Subtle Energy

John Davidson M.A. Cantab.

SAFFRON WALDEN
THE C.W. DANIEL COMPANY LIMITED

First published in Great Britain in 1987 by The C. W. Daniel
Company Limited, 1 Church Path, Saffron Walden,
Essex CB10 1JP, England

ISBN 0 85207 184 1

Production in association with
Book Production Consultants, Cambridge, England
Typeset by Cambridge Photosetting Services in Bembo
Printed and bound by Billings, Worcester

Dedication

This book is dedicated to all of us who share this planet, whatever our caste, creed, position or colour of skin. Putting aside prejudice, let us never abandon the quest for deeper understanding.

'Just as the mind can see that all matter is energy, so the spirit can see that all energy is Love.'

Juan Mascaro, Introduction to the
Bhagavad Gita, Penguin Classics.

'Bold ideas, unjustified anticipations, and speculative thought, are our only means for interpreting nature.'

Sir Karl Popper,
'*The Logic of Scientific Discovery*.

Acknowledgements

A considerable portion of the material for the prologue and the first chapter has been drawn from the literature of the Radha Soami Satsang Beas and from many discussions with fellow followers of this philosophy. In some instances, the sources have been quoted verbatim and credit given accordingly. A full bibliography of sources is given at the end of the book. In other cases, the essence has been extracted while the source has not been mentioned. These two sections rely heavily on the research and writings of Mrs Flora Wood, whose understanding of esoteric matters goes beyond academic description, following a lifetime of study and spiritual practice. I am also grateful to her for going through the manuscript, making a number of valuable suggestions.

There are many folk who have helped directly or indirectly in the production of the remainder of this book. To them, my thanks are due. Marie-Michelle Bailey and Sheila Clark typed and edited the manuscript innumerable times (thank the Lord for word processors!). My wife Farida's pre-print copy has been so well used it looks heavily sat upon, and she has given much support in many ways. When writing the section on homoeopathic miasms, I had a number of fruitful discussions with Roger Savage, whilst Dr George Yao's understanding and explanations of subtle energies have also proved to be of considerable value. Alan Hext – my acupuncturist – got a bimonthly, chapter by chapter account (while I was supposed to be lying in relaxation on his couch) and he fed in many helpful ideas and insights, while Sue Evans, Pat Walsh, Ivor Perry, Roya Bahari and many more of Farida's Iridology students all participated in valuable discussions, raising stimulating ideas. My thanks are also due to Simon Martin who took time from his work as editor and journalist to produce a well-considered foreword and to my publisher, Ian Miller, whose sense of humour has kept me going, while he gradually watched the book turn into something quite different to that which he originally thought he had agreed to publish.

I am grateful to the following authors and/or their publishers for permission to use their copyright:

Fritjof Capra – *The Tao of Physics*

Sylvia Collier – *Canonsburg*, Observer, March 10th, 1985

Davis and Rawls – *The Magnetic Effect*

Davis and Rawls – *Magnetism and Its Effect on The Living System*

John Evans – *Mind, Body and Electromagnetism*

T.C. Lethbridge – *The Power of the Pendulum*

Juan Mascaro – *Introduction to the Bhagavad Gita*

R.P. Aug. Ponlain – *The Mystic Experiences of Medieval Saints*, Kegan Paul

Lowell Ponte – *The Menace of Electric Smog*

Sir Karl Popper – *The Logic of Scientific Discovery*

Radha Soami Satsang Beas – *The Path of the Masters, The Master Answers, Spiritual Gems, The Mystic Bible*

George Sandwith – *Eyewitness to Shamanism*, The Ley Hunter.

Anthony Scott-Morley – *Geopathic Stress, The Reason Why Therapies Fail?*

Dr Randolph Stone – *Health Building – The Conscious Art of Living Well*

Dale Walker – *The Crystal Book*

Lyall Watson – *Supernature*

Paramhansa Yogananda – *Autobiography of a Yogi*

Contents

Foreword

by Simon Martin

Simon Martin is both author and journalist. Probably one of the youngest editors of a major national magazine, he was editor of Here's Health *from 1980–1983, later becoming the founding editor of the successful* Journal of Alternative Medicine. *He is now working as an independent writer on all aspects of health promotion.*

The story behind the writing of this book is like one of those delightful anecdotes that spin out from a practitioners' case history, only in it the 'patient' is John Davidson and I'm a storyteller, not a therapist.

In natural health circles, John and Farida Davidson are well-known for their integrity and their vision. John had formed a research company whilst also working full-time at Cambridge University. At the same time, he was also struggling, unknowingly, with the damaging effects of years of intimate working within the electromagnetic fields and emissions associated with computers.

Through his detailed academic and practical work in the field of what he has termed 'Vibrational Science', John discovered first-hand the stultifying effects on the human complex of pervasive electromagnetic pollution. Luckily, he had also found some answers – spiritually first, I believe, many years previously – later discovering practical ways of combating the drain on his subtle energy banks.

Although creative during his University years, since relinquishing his post in October 1984, John has developed further into someone who is now both solid, sensitive and incredibly productive. This book is evidence of the practical nature of what, at first sight, may seem to be somewhat ethereal.

The book's opening section deals with the philosophy behind the practicalities. Personally, I don't relate to Eastern philosophy too well. When I told him, John said, 'To be complete the story has to start with the Source. Otherwise it would be like trying to describe the planetary orbits without mentioning the sun.' However, the book is mostly about these 'planetary orbits'.

Over the many months he has been writing this book, John has got used to seeing and hearing sections of it coming back at him, in the words and writings of other researchers, but he has never stopped sharing his work with anybody who seemed to be in need of it. Looking for practical ways to use what he was piecing together led him to pioneer the use of Pulsors® in this country. I included some information about these protective devices in an article on electromagnetic pollution I wrote for 'Here's Health' magazine. It was obvious from the article that we were heading into the same area and had reached many of the same conclusions, and on that basis he invited me to write the foreword to his book.

It seems that never before have we had access to so much information about the way our bodies and minds work. Not so long ago, such information was secret, coded for the understanding of an elite. Knowledge is power, and today medical and other professions still retain the vestiges of this self-protective eliteness. In medicine, this is apparent in the use of an arcane language, terminology and technology and the maintenance of a professional mystique.

In medicine and in science, the status of the established elite is maintained by peer pressure to publish research in obscure journals and not to release information to the 'unqualified' before the elite has had a chance to thoroughly acquaint itself with the new knowledge and decide upon a way of making it available.

In practice, this means that there can be a 60-year gap before a potentially life-saving breakthrough becomes routine practice – an institutionalized time lapse that under many circumstances is only shortened when there is personal or commercial profit in it. This is 'old paradigm' science. The 'new paradigm' science recognises that nobody owns truth, least of all those who have a personal interest in concealing it. This new paradigm also recognises that major scientific breakthroughs have often been made by people working outside the areas their training 'allows', who as a result have been castigated as 'amateurs' and have seen their discoveries ignored.

We already have more than enough information to absolutely transform our lifestyles, our health, and the planet who supports us, so that we can achieve the high evolutionary purpose I believe we are here for. The problem is not a lack of information; the problem is a lack of people who can synthesize vast amounts of information, add it up and then simplify it for mass communication.

Not many people have the peculiar sort of mind and the propensity to become instantly energized when on the trail of an extremely odd, anomalous fact that everybody else assures you is irrelevant. I have that sort of mind, and it gladdened my heart to read John Davidson's book (in several stages of its growth), because I realised that he has, too. Not only that, but he has synthesized such a collection of research and practical experience of his own and other people's, that he has probably saved me and other hunter-gatherers several years reading!

John is not only a scientist by training, but has also grown into a sensitive therapist and teacher, so as this book heads from ancient Hindu teaching to Paracelsus, Burr, Reich, polarity and beyond, he is continually striving to make it *practical*.

I have learnt much from this book; I now know how to protect myself from the draining effects of hours of word-processing; and John has generously pushed me into several key areas of reading and research.

In particular, I have become conscious of the crucial role that subtle energy reactions between human and environment play in health and illness, and in the remainder of this introduction, I will suggest ways in which the insights of Vibrational Science will increasingly be used in medicine and healing.

You'd have to be a recluse not to be asking yourself the question, 'What's happening to us?' Violent crime stalks the streets. A nation of animal-lovers, we are now mistreating cats, dogs and horses in horrifying numbers, says the RSPCA.

We are deliberately cruel to the animals we slaughter and eat. What we don't eat we experiment on. If you believe the media reports, most males of our species are drunken, murdering, rapists whose spare-time hobbies include baby-battering and wife-beating.

It's easy to blame the state of humanity on alcohol, junk food and unemployment. Unfortunately, in real life, things aren't that simple.

According to Andrew M. Davie of the Scottish company Geo-Rheological Surveys, criminals aren't really responsible for their actions. He has been able to predict where outbreaks of violence and crime will occur. He's even been able to supply descriptions of the criminals *in advance* of whatever they've got up to.

Similarly, it has been shown as possible to predict, by mathematical survey, where 'accidental' death is likely to develop. 'Cancer houses', for instance, can be pinpointed, as can the time and place of a heart attack, or where there is going to be a spontaneous fire.

Such knowledge is not esoteric, or occult. It was known in ages past and is now being rediscovered. The 'lost' information on which such discoveries as these are based is gradually being pieced together by modern researchers, most of whom figure in this book. And it calls for a drastic reappraisal of our view of ourselves and our world.

One of the main 'unknown' (or uncommunicated) facts is that there are at least two planetary networks of electro-magnetic or perhaps more subtle radiation, about which we already have knowledge: the Curry Grid and the Hartmann Net. The Hartmann Net is something like a giant series of noughts and crosses grids. The Curry Grid is similar, only diagonal. Wherever you have intersections in the Hartmann Net, you get a build up of negative energy and that means trouble. If the intersection is also crossed by a Curry line, then you get an even higher concentration of disharmonizing forces. (See chapter 8).

So if you live or work in a building on one of these intersections, then you have a problem. It doesn't mean that you are going to die young, or commit a crime, although it does seem as if the energy 'pulses' down the grids and nets and may occur at specific intervals.

This may have something to do with solar flares, for

instance, which are known to have a major eleven-year cycle – and there are many 'sunspots' that can be active at any one time. When a sunspot flares, it sends a stream of electromagnetic radiation towards earth, which can affect the climate, especially in regard to its electrical aspects. But the cyclic surges in earth energies that may be caused by these sunspots may also result in freak storms, earthquakes and so on.

So with such 'discoveries' of modern science now revealed to one and all, we have to respect the importance placed on astronomy and astrology by those that were here before us. It is easy to see why observatories and calendars such as Stonehenge were so important, especially when one realises that such stone machines were sited on major lines of energy on the planet's surface. It's not hard to imagine these lines pulsing with energy at different time of the year – and research with geiger counters and electromagnetic radiation recorders at the Rollright stones and other sites have indeed revealed what seems to be cyclical bursts of activity.

The problem nowadays is that we are destroying everything that used to balance out the effects of these pulses of electromagnetic and more subtle energy and protect us from geological radiation – trees, for instance, or running water which is fenced off or polluted to a sludge. Open countryside is rapidly disappearing under buildings and concrete. And to this, we add man-made energy disturbances – power cables, microwave radar, radio and TV broadcasting and so on.

So if you're living in a tower block, in a nearly windowless environment, surrounded by concrete, in polluted air and unnatural light, battered by noise, slumped for hours before a (radiating) TV, eating a junk food diet, smoking *and* drinking too much because you're tense – because you've got people living right on top of you all the time – *and* your home happens to be slap on the intersection of Hartmann and Curry lines, *and* you're a bit upset because you hate your job but you have to do it, and just then there is solar activity releasing a burst of radiation right down the grids (just like electricity through the National Grid), then God knows what you might do.

On the face of it, there's no real reason why an energy we can't see, some of it running through the ground and a great deal more constantly bombarding us in the atmosphere, should make us ill. But as John Davidson shows, while some of the effects are directly physical, measurable and obvious, a lot of them are not. A great deal is to do with the electromagnetic and subtle energies that we have in and around our physical body – the aura, for want of a better word.

It's obvious that matter follows energy – that the physical follows thought. Everything exists as thought first. Take the chair you are sitting on, for instance. Someone had to have the idea of a chair in the first place, they had to visualise what it would look like and what it could do, then eventually it appeared as a physical object.

In an even deeper and more real way, the same is true for the body. As long as you keep your personal force field harmoniously vibrant and intact, you won't have any physical problems. The trouble is that we're living in an atmosphere saturated with radio waves, TV waves, microwaves and so on. So we're already at a disadvantage, then along come other doses of electromagnetic or more subtle energies and blow great holes in the aura. And if you get a disturbance in the aura, the biophysical blueprint, then eventually you will manifest symptoms.

Think about a heart attack, for example, where you get a very clear idea of energy being blocked; or the blocked 'hole' or vortex in the energy field that manifests as a tumour.

We knew that this seemed logical, but until now we did not have much idea about how a disturbance in the subtle energy body could produce the changes at a cellular level that lead to pathology – to symptoms. With John Davidson's synthesis we can begin to see that polarity – the correct balance of positive, negative and neutral – is crucial, and we can see how this polarity has to be maintained at every level: in the energy body, in the subtle energy nervous system of the chakras, through to the physical body via the endocrine system and the physical nervous system and on down to the blood and cells – at every level.

Why, after all, did ancient writings place so much importance on the blood? Why, through the ages, has it been such a symbol of life? Authorities from the nature cure pioneers to modern explorers such as David Tansley maintain that blood is the carrier of life force, which is subtly different from, and at a deeper level of vibration than electromagnetic energy.

In this book we are led to appreciate the significance of the blood afresh. We know that some bacteria in the blood are magnetically active. They are attracted to the site of a cut, for instance, by a change in polarity, 'waking up' and providing a useful role in the process of clotting. And German research has shown that blood clotting is slower in areas of geopathic stress.

So we can begin to appreciate that we are affected by a massive network of influences. We have a planet crisscrossed by grids of electromagnetic and subtle forces; there are underground and overground rivers and streams that have an association with energy flow. We have cyclical 'pulses' in the earth's energy field, caused for instance by sun-spot activity, by the positions of the planets and stars and so on. We can even stir in the possibility that disturbances in the planet's own protective 'aura' can let in 'diseases from space' – as postulated by Sir Fred Hoyle and Chandra Wickramasinghe – bacteria and viruses infiltrating our system from outside the planet's atmosphere.

At this point, we have a choice of interventions: we can plot the likely areas of geopathic disturbance through site and survey dowsing, or mathematically according to Catastrophe Theory and our precise knowledge of the position of the earth's energy grid. We can 'treat' using Feng Shui and other methods of energy harmonization, or we can prevent much of the problem with correct application and understanding of the biological and ecological aspects of buildings. We can also get advance warning of possible cyclical disturbances through the study of both astronomy and astrology.

Then, we can monitor the effects of our increasingly gross interventions in the atmosphere due to nuclear testing, fluorocarbons, carbon dioxide build up, heavy use of other weapons – which, while also catastrophic, are being allowed to proliferate almost in relief that they are non-nuclear. We can also decide to check the sources of electromagnetic pollution that keep our personal energy systems at permanent red alert.

If treatment or prevention is unsuccessful, the cyclical or rhythmical disturbances automatically affect 'homo electronicus' (as Prof. Sedlak of Poland calls modern man) through action on the human being's personal energy field. At this stage, physical illness is still only a potentiality and is open to diagnosis in advance by dowsing and its electronic similars, by instruments of the original Kirlian type, and by the natural or trained sensitivity of other humans.

Here the intervention possibilities become a little more personal. It seems likely that healing, colour therapy, bioelectronic regulatory medicine, meditation, music and visualisation could all significantly alter the otherwise inevitable outcome.

If still unchecked, the subtle energy disturbances lead to changes at a cellular and biochemical – including endocrine – level through an interlocking web of complex 'which comes first – the chicken or the egg?' circumstances. What happens next may depend on whether the blood and the immune system is electrically or magnetically 'tuned' – as a new diagnostic test in Germany suggests. Remember that blood, or whatever it carries, goes *everywhere* in the human complex.

It seems possible that bacterial activity in the blood, both the established, the guessed at, and the relatively newly discovered (see Swedish researcher Dr Erik Enby's work, *Journal of Alternative Medicine*, March, 1986), is an important part of the chain reaction. The focus for disease may well be at a particular site in the body 'prepared' by genetic weakness, environmental action, or straightforward trauma – for example, the documented cases of Poliomyelitis in vaccinated children that always seemed to focus at the site of the needle injury, or at the location of a tonsilectomy or apendectomy, (see Leon Chaitow's new book on vaccination, currently in preparation).

At this stage, depending upon the awareness of the individual, intervention can still be relatively painless. Changes can be made in the environment and lifestyle that is fostering and being fostered by the illness – detoxification, cleansing, nutrition, bacterial re-balancing, for example. We can bring in any of the alternative therapies: homoeopathy, herbal medicine, fasting, hydrotherapy, acupuncture, manipulation, for instance, which clearly act in varying degrees either directly on or around the focus of attack, or indirectly, by reinstating the integrity of the individual's energy field.

The next stage of decline is gross pathology and biological tissue degeneration – the world of tumours and drastic and apparently irreversible physical changes. Yet we know that all these conditions can be reversed. The Gerson Therapy, for instance, a powerful nutritional approach, builds vital force while changing the acid–alkaline balance of the blood.

Even when disease has been allowed to progress to this stage, experience with so-called, alternative therapies prove that it can not only be stopped, but reversed. But amongst allopathic medical therapy, some studies on cancer patients have attempted to demonstrate that effectiveness of therapy is directly related to the personality of the patient because conventional cancer treatment is so hit and miss, despite the millions of pounds spent on securing jobs in researching it.

Yet, no orthodox cancer specialist in this country would even consider telling a patient to change the position of their bed or to protect themselves from electromagnetic pollution. Yet as evidence in this book shows, such simple measures could have dramatic effects.

Then, as I was writing this introduction, came another startling confirmation of the solid basis of the experiments and the hypotheses that John Davidson introduces in his book. My co-worker Cheryl Issacson arrived fresh from the USA with a copy of the American magazine, *Discover*. The front cover story reads:

ELECTRIC MAN

Dr Bjorn Nordenstrom claims to have found in the human body a heretofore unknown universe of electrical activity that's the very foundation of the healing process and is as critical to well-being as the flow of blood.
If he's right, he has made the most profound biomedical discovery of the century.

Inside, a thirteen page article details how Nordenstrom has discovered electrical *polarities* in the bloodstream and how he is manipulating the natural electrical circuits he has found, to disperse tumours!

In the light of what you are about to read in this book, Nordenstrom's discoveries will come as no surprise. When you have read the book, you will probably also not be surprised to learn that Nordenstom's findings have been completely ignored by the vast majority of his colleagues and also by the medical profession.

And this despite the fact that he is a brilliant scientist, who reached the undeniable top of his profession – radiology – as head of diagnostic radiology at Stockholm's Karolinska Institute, was chairman of the Karolinska Nobel Assembly, which chooses the Nobel Prize winner in medicine, and invented a series of radiological practices that were dismissed as too radical in the 1950's but are now in worldwide, routine use.

Nordenstrom is lucky just to have been ignored; as John Davidson shows, many other pioneers in 'Vibrational Science' have been condemned and imprisoned for daring to challenge the establishment. Yet their ideas have survived, waiting for opportunities like this to surface. ... so now read on...

Simon Martin
London, May 1986

Introduction

Our human race is undergoing times of extreme polarity. On the one hand, the development of advanced weaponry based on a little knowledge of the energy structure of matter has made it possible to destroy ourselves and all life on this planet. On the other hand, a new awareness, sensitivity and consciousness is emerging spontaneously amongst the peoples in all parts of our world.

It is expressed at its simplest level by an international cry for environmental consciousness and care, and in its personal form by a developing inner awareness of the mystic and the subtle. It is from here, for example, that much of the surge towards Alternative Medicine takes its roots and its strength.

This polarity, this co-existence of extremes, is indeed a great suffering. But suffering, if undergone with patience and understanding, can give rise to increased humanity, warmth, love and a higher state of being. If indulged in unconsciously, with anger, bitterness and discord, it can end in destruction – in domestic feuds, in suicide, in warfare.

We are, therefore, at a crossroads, in a time of turmoil. There is a surging of energy, a whirling of forces that, as we slowly break through, will give rise to the New Age, a time of greater peace and harmony. Gold needs to undergo the torment of fire, before its inate purity is revealed.

Mystic knowledge and modern physics are now able to meet with understanding. The one representing pure subjective, personal understanding; the other an objective reflection of human thought upon our physical universe. New Age Science combines the inner and the outer in its search for a knowledge of natural forces and how to harness and work with them for man's betterment.

There are many wonders to be revealed in the sub-atomic and more subtle energy fields and new, safe ways of harnessing this energy are yet to be found.

It is from this standpoint that my book: *Subtle Energy* has its roots.

It is inherent in a book of this nature that the future will prove certain statements or conjectures to be correct while other aspects may turn out to be either misguided or simply incomplete. But this book is just an adventure, so the reader should not judge too harshly anything with which they happen to disagree or find difficult to accept. It is necessary to knock before any door will be opened and – according to the intuitions of his inner being and the idiom of the times – the writer is just another human being trying to understand what it's all about.

John Davidson
Cambridge, November 1984

The Mystic Reality

The Perennial Philosophy

Human beings – and all living creatures – are an enigma. We do not know where we came from at our birth, neither do we know what happens at our death. We are thrown about during the years of our life, feeling that we have a separate free-will and identity, despite the fact that rationally we know that we do not even have knowledge of what will happen to us in the next five minutes! We find ourselves, therefore, in a continual paradox.

We have intelligence: consciously or unconsciously, we attempt to unravel the mystery of our existence. Our inner thoughts and feelings reflecting on our outer sensory experience seek understanding. Our minds create explanations of our existence in terms of philosophy, science and religion, but yet we are still not satisfied by their answers. We go on thinking. We cannot stop!

Our mode of thinking, too, is largely a matter of geography, environment and family background. If it had been possible to find an Ultimate Explanation expressed through thoughts and words, it would surely have been found and universally accepted by now.

Is there then a solution to our puzzle? Or is everything pure chaos? Is thinking the correct approach to solving the problem? What, after all, are our thoughts, our mind and our emotions? Even if we were able to spin out the most beautiful philosophy that convincingly covered all aspects of our experience and existence, if that philosophy were expressed in terms of thought alone, the question still arises: what are thoughts? If that cannot be answered, then the whole edifice of the philosophy is suspect. And an explanation of thought by thought is clearly unsatisfactory... This mechanistic and outward approach, therefore, towards understanding our existence will not find the final Cause. It will only describe relationships. It will fit together a few of the pieces in the jigsaw puzzle, but cannot, inherently, form a complete picture. We are ourselves a piece of the puzzle. How can the piece understand the whole puzzle? How can it claim such a freedom?

A good philosophy or scientific theory, therefore, will be one that fits a lot of pieces together. A poor philosophy will ride over logical difficulties with dogma, requiring blind belief of ideas where a rational explanation or the possibility of personal, direct experience, is lacking.

Is there then an alternative approach? Throughout all the complexities of thought along the ages, there has run a strand of simplicity: the simplicity of an inner, totally subjective, mystic experience that transcends matter, time and thought revealing a cosmic pattern and process that cannot be adequately described in outward language.

The inability to describe the experience by anything more than analogy, coupled with a greater or lesser natural distrust of each other, leads those who have never had any inkling of such an experience to incredulity. We cannot experience the feelings and way of being of another fellow human – even his or her day-to-day life – but we can compare their descriptions with our own experience and communication can take place. But if the experience they describe is way out of our experience, we are left with no handle by which to begin to grasp it. At best, we can keep an open mind; at worst, we persecute those who suggest the existence of something of which we are unaware. Indeed, the human race has a history of persecuting those who even *think* differently, let alone those who claim an experience outside our own.

A starting point of honesty has to be reached – a conscious realization that we just do not know what is going on! We are just lost; wandering about between the cradle and the grave, doing our best, which may even be our worst!

Everybody has an inner life and an outer life. The outer life is inherently complex, the inner life of most of us is even more so. In fact, we have only one life, one existence – our outer life is simply an expression of our inner life. There is, really, no truly objective experience, something separate from us. As soon as we begin to think about a thing, it becomes a part of our subjective experience. Even our sensory perceptions of the world are experienced within ourselves, The world we think to be outside us is really within us: we experience it, outside, from within ourselves.

It is all a question of the direction of our attention. When our attention is directed outside, we feel that the world is outside and separate from us. When the attention is directed within, in specific meditational or spiritual practices, then a whole new world of being begins to open to us. We feel like one who is slowly awakening from a vivid dream. The dream goes on, but our understanding of its relative reality and importance changes.

This philosophy of an inner experience of the nature of Reality is as old as man. It has been called the Perennial Philosophy. It springs spontaneously from the inner experience of individuals in cultures widely separate and who have had no communication with each other. This experience is powerful enough to be the mainspring from which all world religions are later derived, after the death of those who had the experience. These people we call Mystics. The highest mystic experience is described as one of Love, Light and Supreme Understanding: of merging, inwardly, with the Source of Being and becoming One with it.

This Source is known by a myriad names and in all languages: Supreme Being, Universal Consciousness, God, Reality. There are many inspiring books which trace this philosophy through the ages.

Wherever access to the original philosophy of these Mystics is available, we find insistence on the practice of meditation, of spiritual disciplines designed to prepare and awaken the inner nature of man to move towards this experience. We find, too, a cosmology which places our physical world as a hair in an ocean of a heirachy of inner worlds accessible within man and out of which our physical universe is derived.

The Mystic Cosmology

All mystics and mystic philosophies agree that there is one Source, one central self-sustaining Powerhouse of Consciousness and pure Being. From this Source, a hierarchy of worlds – the Creation – have their existence as an emanation or projection from the Source, providing a continuum of stepped-down energies that are the basis for this hierarchy and the beings or souls who inhabit its various regions. In Vedic terminology, (the Vedas are ancient Hindu writings), the word used is *Leela* or 'play'. The ancient sages say that the creation is just the play or projection of the Creator. It is His game of Love.

There is, say the mystics, nothing but the Supreme Being or Consciousness: all individual souls are drops in that Ocean. All inanimate mind, matter and energy are a part of That. There is nothing but the One. If there was something else besides, He would not be the One. Everything is contained within Him.

Mystics have called this Great ubiquitous Power by a multitude of names that reflect the many attitudes and concepts we human beings are able to accept or understand concerning Him or It. He is One and Nameless, mystics call Him by many names. Our planet is inhabited by a myriad of humans who, although essentially the same in basic mental and physical characteristics, all express themselves differently and have varying customs and cultures. This is self-evident, but just like a couple who want to live harmoniously, but always end up fighting, our ways of thinking give us preferences and prejudices around which we find it difficult to see. Amongst people, therefore, who intuitively understand the basics of spiritual or mystic philosophy, their manner of expression and favoured terminology varies. Some prefer to talk of the Universal Consciousness, others like the more personal approach of God, the Lord, the Father.

The Reality is One, and men also call It by different names. I can remember a time, some years ago, when a natural negative reaction to a conventional, 'religious' upbringing, made it impossible for me to consider calling the Source as God. And this was true, for the way God had been described by conventional Christianity was so far removed from the mystic Power of my later understanding that the meaning conditioned in me of the word 'God' was quite different.

Now, with the passage of time, the old meaning has almost been lost, and I can use most terminology without feelings of reservation. Generally, when speaking cos-mologically, one considers the One as the Universal Source or Supreme Being. When thinking personally, He is the Lord whose attribute is Love and into whom the drop of one's own being is in the process of merging.

So one should not be over-analytical of words, but look beyond them, to the meaning. In the *Book of Mirdad*, the author says: 'Words are at best an honest lie'. With words, we can at best only give honest indications of our thoughts and way of being: we cannot transmit the background to why we think and feel the way we do or what our inner being is really feeling or experiencing.

All mystic philosophies, then, have described a cosmol-ogy in which everything is created from within itself. Mystics have all said that this entire physical universe is no larger than a hair in comparison to the immensity of the inner worlds. These inner worlds have their own activities and inhabitants and the soul is active there through a body of these same energy vibrations.

In terms of energy, therefore, we have a closed system in which everything lives and moves and has its being. This includes the energy of our own thought and consciousness.

From our human point of view, looking horizontally or outwardly at the physical world from within a physical body, we can provide descriptions at the physical level. From a universal point of view, looking vertically or inwards, we find that the physical universe is a reflection downwards of energy vibrations from more subtle worlds, which are, in turn, reflections of more inner or subtle worlds or energy fields.

Creation or existence, then, is a stepping down or a progression outwards from the Source. It is also a continu-ous and dynamic process.

Mystics say that, although the energy progression out-wards from the centre represents a continuum, there are specific points that may be termed energy crossroads or focus points. These are the centres of power or energy distribution, such as the chakras of the physical body. The only way to really understand this, is, of course, to experi-ence it, but descriptions and philosophies are relevant, being of importance to us as humans, so we may continue.

Thus it is that a specific cosmology is described in terms of physical, astral, causal and spiritual planes, with their corresponding bodies, through which the individual soul operates in these planes or levels of consciousness. However, because of the immensity of the inner worlds and because particular mystics themselves may not have reached to the Source, but perhaps only a little way above our physical world, there are a variety of cosmologies given to us by different mystics, depending on their particular inner experiences. The variations in their descriptions do not invalidate the reports of all such experiences any more than the variations in descriptions of the things of this world disprove their existence. Furthermore, much of the present day literature regarding these topics is *not written from first hand experience*, but from descriptions found by the authors in a variety of places and taken from a multitude of, often unknown, sources.

In addition, the vastness of the inner realms is literally beyond imagination and inferences drawn from the experiences of one mystic are likely to be different in content to that described by another; just as descriptions, by different people, of the American and European continents on this earth will have certain similarities, but also some essential and valid differences.

Finally, just as two visitors to the same place in this world will describe it differently, so also will mystics describe their essentially indescribable experience in varying terms according to their own background, as well as that of their audience.

All mystics agree on one point, however, and that is the existence of the one Source of Being of which everything else is a reflection or projection. Furthermore, they all state that this Being is not far away, but that It is an inherent part of us and is 'closer than breathing, nearer than hands and feet'. Indeed, He is within us, at the heart of our being. He is an Ocean of Love, Light, Bliss and Consciousness – Pure Being. We are drops in that Ocean. A true mystic or realized soul of the highest order is one who has been drawn into that Ocean and become one with it.

With this in mind, therefore, let us briefly describe the mystic cosmology from the highest to the lowest aspects of creation. The remainder of the book is then concerned primarily with the physical and subtle physical aspects –

with the inch or two of which we are all more or less aware and which lies at the bottom of this ten thousand mile journey within our own beings. But, says Confuscius, a ten thousand mile journey starts with the first step.

A true mystic cosmology is both the simple and profound. It will have within it, a place of non-critical understanding for all other cosmologies and philosophies. Inasmuch as answers can be given, it will have an answer to everything, both spiritual and mundane. Most importantly, the emphasis will be on specific spiritual disciplines and meditation as described by a living and loving, present day mystic, to experience the truth of the cosmology at first hand. It will not be an intellectual philosophy; it will be a practical path of spiritual development.

No ritual or dogma will be involved. Practitioners will be required to believe nothing blindly, but simply to take the philosophical aspects as a working hypothesis and follow the spiritual disciplines prescribed in order to prove (or disprove) by experience inwardly, the validity of the outer philosophy and description. No money will be solicited from followers, nor would they be required to change their dress or mode of living other than is required by decent standards of morality and good social behaviour. Such a philosophy would be totally inward, with no proseletization or unnecessary, outward trappings.

Such a mystic philosophy is not new. In fact, it is as old as man and as natural as being alive. In this description, I have used Hindi and Sanskrit terminology, because there are usually no clear parallels in the English language. Where English parallels are available I have used them, attempting at the same time to point out that words such as 'astral' and 'causal', for example, are used so loosely and confusingly in most writings on mystical subjects as to be more a hindrance than a help to clarity. There is no reason in modern times for mystic writings to be veiled in symbolism or shrouded in a cloak of 'occulty wish-wash'. Actually, this often obscures a lack of knowledge on the part of the writer who may be writing only from hearsay or without adequate guidance.

According to the deepest mystic philosophy, in the region of the highest, there exists no duality or separateness. In an Ocean of Love, all is One. That One is nameless, formless and inaccessible. Names and forms exist only when there is differentiation and separateness. The individual, as an individual, can have no access, but must first lose all trace of I-ness and become the One.

From this highest, comes an outpouring of creative *energy*: the *Word*, the *Life Stream*, the *Will of the Supreme*. It is known by numerous names throughout the cultures of the world. In Hindi, it is called *Adi Shabd*. Journeying forth, this Power takes on the first 'form', known as *Sat Purush* (True Being) and rests in the first region, *Sat Lok* (True Location). On every occasion in its downward journey where it rests (downward, not in terms of space, but in the quality of vibration) a succession of areas of power arise, each with their nuclei: which we may call *regions*, with their governors; their extent being vast. Christ spoke of them, saying: 'In my Father's house are many mansions'.

These two streams of power, Sat Purush and Adi Shabd go further and create another location, called *Par Brahm*, consisting of spirit only tenuously permeated by a highly refined, primal thought form, a 'side-effect' brought about by their movement and called *Prakriti* (primal matter). The current so created here is known as *Akshar Purush*.

Par Brahm consists of two characteristic areas, the higher of which is known as *Bhanwar Gupha* (the Whirling Cave), the need for movement being caused by the vast will of the power to create and project downwards. The three currents of Sat Purush, Adi Shabd and Akshar Purush, here draw together at a point known as *Tribeni* (three rivers or currents) and like the centre of a whirlpool draw downwards in a tunnel-like form, leading into the lower area of Par Brahm known as *Daswan Dwar*.

These tunnels of downward projection differentiate one region from another like valves with an easy flow downwards, but very difficult for re-entry in reverse. This first tunnel is known as *Maha Sunna* (the Great Void) and is of an unplumbed depth and an intense darkness. It represents the final barrier of the soul from the Source. Only by the Will of the Supreme and in the companionship of a true saint, can it be crossed.

The power then flows out into a vast reservoir of energy called *Mansarovar*. From here, the three streams of energy again flow together through a channel known as the *Tenth*

Door, leaving the realm where spirit predominates to enter the confines of the *Universal Mind* or *Brahm*, also known as *Kal*.

As the soul descends below Daswan Dwar, something of tremendous significance takes place: the soul takes on the first coverings of the mind in order to communicate with, and operate in the realm of Brahm, Kal or Universal Mind, also known as the causal region. Above Brahm, the soul is naked and knows itself as soul. Our true being is soul or consciousness, mind is inanimate and takes its existence from the soul. Just as the physical body is inanimate matter, but is maintained in existence through the presence of our life force within it, so also is the mind 'dead', taking its power to move and exist from the spirit or soul.

The Universal Mind is also the region where *Time* is first manifest. It is the region or part of us that is responsible for rationality. The mind is a super-computer whose overriding law is cause and effect or justice, also called *Karma*, in Hindu terminology.

From here on down, everything happens due to cause and effect. Above this region, the prevailing law is Love, unity, merging.

The soul, in this region, takes on a causal body and a corresponding causal mind in order to function here. The cloak of the causal coverings is so subtle that those mystics ascending to this point have often confused it with the final Source and have declared that the universe is the creation of Universal Mind. They are correct, but have not reached to the Source of the Universal Mind to know that the Universal Mind is also a creation and not the absolute and eternal.

The attributes of these regions are *Light* and *Sound* manifesting as subtle and beautiful forms and bodies analogous to, but far surpassing, those of our physical world. The inner being of the souls in these regions is steeped in deep bliss, love and peace.

The three streams of Sat Purush, Adi Shabd and Akshar Purush flow out into the higher confines of *Brahmand* (the region of Brahm, the causal region) to the foot of three eminences or mountains known as *Mer*, *Sumer* and *Kailash*, whose shining peaks give this region its Hindu name of *Trikuti* meaning 'three forts'.

The controlling power, lord or ruler of Trikuti is known

as Brahm or Kal (the Lord of Time) with the receptive pole or female counterpart of *Maya* (Illusion). Maya is the power of concealment and of projection into lower planes. We are now in the world of duality and all positive controlling powers are balanced by a negative or receptive pole. The One has begun its journey into the many.

The externalization of these powers and the loss of their true inner meaning is responsible for the million Gods of Hinduism. The rich, spiritual heritage in the sacred literature of Hinduism, plus the teachings of yogis and mystics of varying degrees of attainment, degenerates, without the personal guidance of a true mystic, into outward rituals, formalities and worship of these powers as deities to be venerated. This degeneration of the teachings of mystics into religious formalities is the characteristic and understandable pathway when the inner meaning and spiritual practice is lost. It is responsible for all the main world religions.

Returning to our description of the energy pathways emanating from the Supreme, in the region of Universal Mind, the first three creative currents are joined by Kal and Maya, making five in all. In fact, it is the movement, the downward creative urge, reacting upon itself that creates all lower powers. Kal and Maya are a creation of the first three currents, just as all currents are emanations from the Supreme. Through the illusive garment which Maya begins to weave around them, creating the illusion of time, space and causation, a sense of separateness is increasingly felt and they give rise to the formation of the three attributes or *gunas*, discussed in all Hindu literature.

The three gunas are:

1. *Rajas Guna*, the attribute of activity, of coming into being, of creation, the positive pole, the motor power, the restless drive of the mind and emotions for action and fulfillment.

2. *Satvas Guna*, the attribute of harmony, of preservation, of peace, the neutral pole.

3. *Tamas Guna*, the attribute of inertia, decay, dissolution, darkness and resistance to all action.

If we look at any aspect of life, we can see these three attributes in action. We can see it in the seasons of the year – in both the annual cycle as well as cycles within cycles; we see them in personalities; in our individual span of life. We see them operating in the mundane, as well as the apparently important.

Furthermore, each guna can have positive and negative activity. There is a right time for creation, a right time for preservation, a right time for dissolution or destruction. We take down an old delapidated building to construct a new one, that is a positive aspect of the tamas guna. Nature too has a time of fall and winter, a time of rest and recuperation.

In Taoist Chinese philosophy, much of which is said to be derived from the ancient Indian cultures, the gunas are known as *Yin* (tamas, receptive, female principle) and *Yang* (rajas, expanding, male principle). Tao is that which cannot be spoken, uttered or described. It is the One or, as the creative principle, it is the Adi Shabd. It is through inner attention to this Shabd or Tao that one follows the Way back to the Source, beyond manifestation. While still within the realms of the gunas or yin and yang, one strives for harmony and balance. This is the satvas guna or harmonious balance of yin and yang, but the ultimate 'goal' lies beyond all opposites and attributes. And, it is said, it is not far away. It is 'nearer than breathing, closer than hands and feet'. It is right within us, indeed it is what constitutes our real essence of being.

Once more, resuming our journey with the energy currents, the now eight currents of Trikuti (three primal plus Kal, Maya and the three gunas) meet the causal state or mental idea of the five *tattwas* or *elements*, the pre-cursors or blueprint of the dense material out of which our physical universe and body are constructed. At this stage, the energy currents of the five tattwas are extremely fine and subtle. The blueprint of the blueprint, so to speak, of our gross physical universe. The five elements or states are:

1. *Prithvi*, Earth or the solid state of matter.

2. *Jal*, Water or liquid state of matter.

3. *Agni*, Fire or the state of heat.

4. *Vayu*, Air or the gaseous state.

5. *Akash*, Ether, the primordial ingredient out of which the universe is created and the other elements have their being. If one can catch the implied meaning, it is also described as 'space' or 'vacuum'.

The first five currents interacting upon the five tattwas produce the twenty five *prakritis*, or conditions of mind and matter. At this level, like the tattwas, they are the energy blueprint of the blueprint of what becomes manifest at the physical level. The twenty five prakritis – not to be confused with Prakriti (primal matter) in Trikuti – are essentially subdivisions of activity within the energy fields of the five tattwas. Thus, at the gross physical level, the earth element has prakritis that cover all the solid aspects of the body – bones, flesh, skin, hair, blood vessels and so on whilst the prakritis associated with the water element govern and provide the subtle material substrate for body fluids – blood, urine, lymph, cytoplasm, exocrine secretions etc. The fire element is associated with more subtle aspects of body management such as hunger and thirst, while the airy and etheric elements consist of essential principles – expansion and contraction (airy qualities) – and mental/emotional attributes such as desire and consciousness of self (etheric attributes).

These categories are only briefly noted and should be taken in a wide context to include all systems and parts of the body. This understanding of the body through the basic elements of which it is constituted is at the basis of the ancient Indian system of healing known as Ayurvedic Medicine. It is the soul or consciousness in the body, acting through the mind and *pranas* or subtle energies that keeps these otherwise 'inimical' energy fields together. At death, when the soul departs, the disintegration of the body and the parting of the elements immediately commences – 'ashes to ashes, dust to dust'. Ayurveda attempts to create harmony (or health) within these vibrating energy fields.

Each of the eight currents in Trikuti attract and absorb the five modifications, prakritis or aspects of the five tattwas, making forty currents in all. Like spinning flames of energy or the petals of a flower chalice, they assume a lotus-like shape. Projecting downwards, the forty energy currents, interacting on the twenty five prakritis, each carrying its own attributes, colours and sounds, all throbbing and glowing with astral effulgence and energy, making a total of one thousand (40 × 25) flame shaped currents, plus one central flame (the origin of the mantra: 'Om mane padme hum' – 'Consider the jewel in the lotus'), create what is known as *Sahansdal Kanwal*, the *Thousand Petalled Lotus*, sometimes called the *Mountain of Light*, the powerhouse of this astral region and the regions below, down to the physical. It is called astral because the faculty of vision is more perfect and that which is seen is brighter than anything upon this earth, brilliant as though seen through a rainbow and shimmering as with star-dust. Each of these flame-shaped jets is the energy responsible for the existence of a portion of the physical universe, drawing its life force from this celestial source.

Causal and astral energies on earth, however, are very weak dilutions of these thousand streams of power, far less subtle and volatile and with a greatly limited range. Through the sub-astral regions below this plane, these thousand currents contrive to act separately and in illimitable permutations and combinations, slowly diminishing in effulgence and energy as they interact, but nevertheless presenting a spectacle of breathtaking beguilement and splendour, vividly dancing and whirling in endless displays.

As matter condenses on them, as they move, they slowly stultify and sink until they are drawn down to create the physical universe as we know it. Like a grand and tragic opera drawing to its close, the music of the primal Adi Shabd or Life Stream is hushed. The diffused and frustrated currents now enter the sphere of the physical human mind with its attributes (*Antashkarans*) of intellect (*Buddhi*), memory (*Chit*), volition and change (*Manas*) and the greatest stumbling block of all, human ego (*Ahankar*).

As the soul comes down through the causal, astral and physical realms, it takes on coverings or bodies in order to be able to communicate and exist at those levels. The prevalent mood of the higher astral levels is of bliss and peace. However, the innate feelings of distress in the soul at being separated by increasing unconsciousness from its source are now felt not so much as an inward and blissful longing, but as a desire to fill the vacuum by activity and motion, both inward and outward, in the energy fields surrounding it. In other words, the attention is moving downwards and outwards towards birth on the physical plane of existence.

Just as an electric current, after leaving the main power-house, has to be reduced at transforming stations, so that it may be dilute enough for domestic consumption, so the great main current of the Life Stream undergoes a change at these localities and becomes clothed in the coats of the various regions through which it passes.

By that first desire, evinced at the top of Brahm, the law of cause and effect, of karma, has associated the Life Stream with time, space, relativity, creation, preservation, destruction, the pairs of opposites, illusion, and all the attributes of the human mind. These have rendered its isolation from its source complete. Indeed, the covering is so effective that the poor soul cannot find its way back through the mass of tiny threads of relationships that bind it to earth. If by good chance it loosens some of its threads, through habit it reassumes thousands more. The souls take birth again and again in the multitude of bodies available in the physical world for the satisfaction of unfulfilled desire and the outworking of the law of karma, cause and effect.

Only a perfect and unencumbered soul, straight from the Source can cut through these threads giving back to the lost soul its inner sight and hearing (*Surat* and *Nirat*) to find its way on to the road back to its original Home in the shortest possible time.

Words are, of course, often a source of confusion when describing these regions and planes of consciousness and there are esoteric schools of thought that describe astral and causal energies as those which in this cosmology are equatable with emotional and mental energies within the lower human constitution. The 'ego body' also mentioned is probably equatable with the *ahankar* in its association with *chit* or 'mind stuff.'

When the mental or astral form of man was first projected from *Anda*, the astral realm, as an isolated soul or *jiva* (a jiva is an unenlightened soul imprisoned in a physical body), the primary substance which at this stage is known as *Akash*, enveloped itself with *Prana* (the force of the Life Stream clothing itself with mind substance – the pattern form, or subtle energy blueprint of the physical body), in order that it might 'live' on earth a part of *Pinda*, the physical plane. This prana plus akash, we understand as 'breath' or 'breathing' on these planes. It takes care of the subconscious acts of living. It is prana, for instance, exerting attraction, of which magnetism and gravity are a part, which, holding matter together, forms the earth or which causes a baby to take its first breath, sets the heart beating and the digestion working, etc.; in other words, vitalizes the whole build-up, maintenance, and break-down of substances within this plane, without any conscious effort on our part.

Akash is a term met frquently in esoteric and yogic literature and can be source of confusion. It also means 'sky' in the sense that all energies are created from above (or within) and like the other elements is found first in seed form in Trikuti or the causal region. Again it is reflected in Sahansdal Kanwal or the true astral region and once again in subtle physical matter in the throat chakra.

The jiva thus clothed itself in a physical form, dictated by the sum-total of its karmas to date. In the earliest stage or days of creation all was fresh, and vital – it was in fact, the *Golden Age (Sat Yuga)*, so all five tattwas were present in this new being; he was 'Man', a balanced personality, with the satvas guna preponderating. However, as act succeeded act (*pralabdh* or destiny karma) in his new life upon earth, with the aid of the five senses working through the nine orifices of the body, (two eyes, two ears, two nostrils, mouth and two lower outlets), the gunas began to go out of balance and either the rajas guna (of excessive action) took command or the tamas guna (of excessive in-action or inertia) asserted itself, and slowly the original primary element of akash was leached away and the jiva began to take on animal characteristics. It therefore became necessary for him to inhabit a type of body in which it was impossible for him to make new or *kryaman* karma, so that he might earn the 'right' to a new stock of akash and, depending on the violence of his swing to right or left (rajas or tamas), so he was given an animal body or a bird, insect, or vegetable body.

In other words, the Golden Age had begun to die, giving place to ages progressively weaker in akash power, i.e. *Silver, Copper* and at the last *Iron*, (*Treta, Dwapar* and *Kal Yugas*). For every step he descended, near or nearer to the earth, he inevitably forfeited one tattwa to suffer a progressively gloomier fate. He, himself, by his own act had pulled the first string that set him dancing like a puppet; but thenceforth each act had reduced his free-will further and further. Sometimes the balance of his karma allowed a little akash tattwa to re-enter his make-up, but this was squandered again rapidly through growing layers of bad habit and down he would go again, with a new load. And this is where we now find ourselves.

Ultimately, the plight of the soul becomes such that the much-inhibited Shabd or Life Stream activating him, sends up a signal to the ocean of Shabd, to the Supreme One, that it is in such hopeless difficulties that only the strongest arm can rescue the jiva. Being all Love, that Creator, that Supreme is moved to intense compassion and projects Himself down through all the layers of His creation, incarnating as a Saviour or Teacher upon the same plane as His child in distress, laying upon Himself all the restraints in which His child (the isolated soul) has become involved. He puts forth His beloved hand and touches the tortured frame of the supplicant. Immediately his strength begins to return, restoring the balance of the tattwas, gunas, etc., so that he is brought back to Man's estate, with the added desire to know God once more a conscious part of his make-up.

Masters have always been present upon earth, but because he was content with his lot, man did not avail himself of their help in the earlier ages. In Kal Yuga, in which we find ourselves at present, akash has become so depleted that life has entered the Dark Ages. Perfect Masters or *Sat Gurus* are actively engaged in teaching upon the physical plane to give eternal relief to suffering, and men eagerly seek their assistance. The total karma of each individual to be regenerated by a Master is brought into a state nearer equilibrium than it has been since its fall, and automatically that person commences seeking for spiritual awakening and release. The isolation of the soul has at last ceased. It has broken through the vicious circle of involvement with the negative planes, is about to turn around facing the light of eternity once more, with the assurance of a return to its original home.

Karma and Reincarnation

Here and there, throughout this book I mention aspects of karma and the associated philosophy of reincarnation, so it makes sense to explain very briefly the basics of this philosophy, though a 'belief' in reincarnation or even the law of karma is not essential to appreciating much of the contents of this book.

Karma means action, or doing. Everything in the physical universe, says this ancient philosophy, happens due to cause and effect. Scientists would not disagree with this, but it is taken a step further. Not only is cause and effect the law of material relationships in this world amongst the horizontal energy spectrum, but it is also the law by which things happen in the vertical energy spectrum.

What this means, in practice, is that all our actions, thoughts, emotions, desires etc. make an impression on the soft wax of our mind; they become a cause, the effect of which is felt in subsequent births. In fact, all the effects or karma – good or bad – of our existence in one life become the substance upon which our next life is based, our destiny, with any karma left over being placed in storage within the complex structure of our higher mind, to be used for better or worse in future lives, or held in storage indefinitely.

Mystics talk of three types of karma. Firstly, our *prahlabd* or destiny karma with which we are born and which governs our basic personality and the major framework of our life. Within that structure, we have a conditioned free-will to perform *kryaman* or new karma. Upon our death, we either spend some time in the inner regions or immediately take another birth, but either way our kryaman karma created in previous lives become our prahlabd karma for future lives with anything left over becoming our *sinchit* or store of unused karma. Our prahlabd karma will also contain karma from our sinchit store, so we are likely to be facing events in one life that relate to many different lives from the past.

There are many aspects to this philosophy that can be brought out, but it is not my intention to do so here. Suffice it to say that nature loses nothing, neither is something created out of nowhere. Unfulfilled desires, the effect of our actions on our own minds and those of others, plus deep grooves in the mind from one life that remain unsatiated or uncleared, will be carried forward to a future life. That energy complex does not just disappear at the death of the body, it has to have an outworking. Tangled and 'uncompleted' relationships with people draw us back to the same people time after time. Christ also says: 'Even the hairs on your head are all numbered' – it means that the law of karma and its inescapable corollary of reincarnation, are inexorable. Our actions to escape are like that of a man caught in quicksand – we simply become further entangled. Only with the help of one who is beyond this churning wheel can we get out of the realm of births and death.

CHAPTER I

The Microcosm and the Macrocosm – The Subtle Constitution of Man

In the prologue, we discussed how in the mystic cosmology, the physical universe is a reflection of the astral and the astral a reflection of the causal. As a part of the integration of these regions within his constitution, a soul has a body made up of the substance of each region. In addition, a reflection or ray of the Universal Mind is also present as the physical, astral and causal minds. Furthermore, man, while in his physical form, has within himself access to the entire universe through centres of energy or *chakras* – distribution and control points for tapping or permitting access to the higher energy vibrations.

The six chakras of the physical body are frequently discussed in esoteric literature. What is not always known is that these chakras are a reflection of the six chakras within the astral body, which in turn are a reflection of the six chakras of the causal body. The characteristics of energy at these reflected centres is similar to their conterparts above and below giving rise to much confusion when understanding the descriptions given by yogis and others, of their experiences, since it is thus possible to feel that one has reached to the top of the Universal Mind while still in fact residing in the astral or even sub-astral regions.

Man is therefore the microcosm, reflecting all stages of the macrocosm within himself and being capable, with guidance and practice, of penetrating the darkness of his earthly consciousness and rising up within himself to the highest level of Pure Being.

In the Hindu Vedas, the Sanskrit word commonly translated as 'creation' is more exactly rendered as 'projection'. The ancient sages, aware that something cannot be created out of nothing, expresssed this inner knowledge when they said that the Supreme One projects Himself into form and material substance. It means that there is nothing but Him.

He is always present within the smallest particle of his creation. His power is manifested as energy stepped down to different vibratory levels corresponding to the different realms of creation, finally reaching the lowest pole of negativity in the physical universe.

This is illustrated by the phenomenon of our physical mind, wherein our thoughts have their being. Manas, buddhi, etc., and all the elements of our physical mind, are simply the projections of the cosmic or Universal Mind, the *Mahat*. This Mahat then becomes manifested in vibrating thought, our human mind with qualities akin to those of the universal. The rationality and logic of our clearest human thought being a reflection or expression of the super-computer logic and controlling law of cause and effect, first manifested in the Universal Mind and operating throughout all lower regions. Nothing is ever created new except as to form. Its substance is as eternal as the Creator Himself, and through everything the creative essence runs.

The Six Chakras Within The Physical Body

We are now in a position to describe the six chakras of the physical body. These chakras lie in subtle energy fields, a part of the physical universe and of the energy blueprint which controls and creates the functions and existence of the gross physical body as we know it.

As with all cosmic energy, they can be experienced in the inner consciousness of man as light and sound. Light and sound, indeed all our senses, represent our ability to perceive vibrations or movement within energy fields – our knowledge of change within the energy patterns that constitute the creation. Each chakra is shaped like a lotus flower with a varying number of petals or energy aspects, a replica of the one thousand petalled lotus of the astral powerhouse, each petal representing an energy current, the interactions between them resulting in the creation of all below.

It is an interesting fact that these body chakras taken together have exactly fifty-two petals, corresponding to the fifty-two letters in the Sanskrit alphabet. Each petal gives out a sound, a distinct vibration or musical note, corresponding to the sound of one of the Sanskrit letters. These sounds can be heard by any person whose finer sense of hearing has been awakened. He can then see these chakras and listen to their sounds. It is said that these fifty-two comprise all the sounds which can possibly be made by the vocal organs of man. They say that the ancient rishis, listening to those fifty-two sounds, fashioned a character for each one, and that is why the Sanskrit language is called *Dev Bani: the Language of the Gods.*

Name	No. of petals	Colour	Position	Element	Endocrine Gland
Ajna	2	White & Black	Between Eyes		Pituitary & Hypothalamus
Kanth	16	Dark Blue	Throat	Akash	Thyroid & Parathyroid
Hriday	12	Blue	Heart	Air	Thymus
Manipurak	8	Dark Red	Solar Plexus	Fire	Pancreas
Svadasthan	6	Whitish-Black	Sacrum	Water	Gonads
Muladhara	4	Reddish	Coccyx	Earth	Adrenals

The Six Chakras Within The Physical Body

Beginning from the lowest chakra:

The *Mul Chakra*, also known as *Muladhara* or *Guda Chakra*, is situated at the back of the rectum and governs elimination. In Hindu terminology, the 'deity' or controlling energy centre of this region is called *Ganesh*, the elephant-headed god who has no female or receptive counterpart. This chakra has four petals or letters, its colour is red and its element is earth or solids (Prithvi). In former times, when practising pranayam or ashtang yoga, the start was ordinarily made from this centre. It was for this reason that amongst the Hindus, the worship of Ganesh is enjoined before undertaking any activity of importance. Hence Ganesh is also looked upon as the god of Good Luck.

The rectal chakra is, in a sense, the base support of the other chakras. With its subtle elemental essence (tattwa) or blueprint being that of the solid or earthy state of matter, it controls and administers those associated aspects of the body – the bones, muscles, skin, hair and blood vessels and so on.

Each chakra is associated with a major endocrine or hormonal gland as part of the pathway by which the inner, vital life energies are externalized or crystallized as observable physical existence. The rectal chakra manifests outwardly through the adrenal glands – the basis of protective activity in our human system.

Attachment to physical objects is the human perversion associated with this chakra and its concomitant – fear – follows as a direct result of this weakness. The desireless person has no attachments and fears nothing, since he knows he has nothing real to lose. Fear is also associated with adrenaline, the fight or flight hormone of the adrenal medulla that prepares one to protect one's existence on this plane. So one can readily see how this chakra plays the role of protector and supporter of gross physical existence.

The second or *Indri Chakra*, also called the *Swada* or *Svadasthan Chakra*, is situated near the sacral plexus and controls the creation of the physical frame, its energy and procreative desires. It has six petals or letters. Its colour is yellow and the names of its Hindu deities are *Brahma* (not to be confused with Brahm, or Universal Mind) and Savitri. The element is water (Jal or Pani) – water being the matrix out of which all living substances evolve in the process of creation, even as the unborn infant floats in the amniotic fluid. Its guna is the creative (rajas). The element of this chakra being water, its energies administer the fluids of the body – blood, lymph, mucus, semen, urine and so on. Its human weakness is that of lust or sensory indulgence of any kind, which pulls the consciousness away from its rational seat behind the eyes. Its energy flows in particular through the gonads also manifesting as the sex hormones oestrogen, progesterone and testosterone, all three being steroids of similar composition and capable of being transformed by the body one into another. Seen as energy vibrations, these molecules are very similar – a point we will return to in a later chapter.

In association with the chakras are the system of *nadis*, a network of subtle 'nerves' or pathways by which *prana* or life energy is distributed throughout the body. Over 72,000 nadis are said to be interwoven within the body, of which three, *Shushumana*, *Pingala* and *Ida*, are of particular importance. *Shushumana* passes through the central spinal canal linking the chakras with each other. Starting on the right of the basal, Mul chakra, runs *Pingala*, whilst on the left lies *Ida*. These two canals or nadis, crossing over left to right as they rise up, reach only as far as the *Do-Dal-Kanwal*, the chakra behind and between the two eyes. From the central nadi, also known as the *Royal Vein* or *Kundalini*, twenty-four smaller nadis or energy channels spring forth, there being ten major channels, five on each side, including Ida and Pingala. The true creative life current, Shabd, which takes the soul up to higher regions, does not descend below the eye centre; below that, its creative and organizational energy is distributed through the medium of the pranas, being finally hushed and lying 'at rest' in the Mul chakra. Here the life force is said to be coiled, meaning thereby that it is energy as potential, stored energy like that in a compressed spring.

The coiling of energy at the base of Shushumana is also known in the Sanskrit literature as Kundalini, concerning which considerable and erroneous speculation has been made in western esoteric literature.

When, through *Pranayama* or other yogic control of the pranas and chakras, the yogi is able to concentrate his attention into each of the chakras and awaken his consciousness to the subtle energies, this potential pranic energy rises up along the Shushumana, (Kundalini is sometimes equated with the Shushumana itself). That is, prana flows freely up the Shushumana, to the eye centre, under the control of the inwardly concentrated attention of the practitioner. This is what has become known as the 'raising of the Kundalini.'

But this practice can take one only as far as the eye centre. For further ascent, it is necessary to take the help of the Light or of the Shabd or Inner Sound. Ultimately, only the Shabd, being the creatve power itself, also manifesting as light, can take the soul to the Source. Mystics of the highest order do speak of the six chakras, so that people may not be confused and think that they do not know about them. But they always advise that spiritual practice should commence at the eye centre and work up from there with the help of the Shabd.

The 'awakening' of the chakras and the pranic currents

inherent in Kundalini or in the Shushumana takes years and years of intense, inner yogic practice. As the centres are awakened or as the practitioner's consciousness penetrates these subtle energy fields, power over the associated tattwas is also realized, giving the yogi the ability to perform miracles – walk on water, fly in the air, sit on fire, manifest objects and so on. In fact, anything projected out of the tattwas comes within his grasp as his consciousness expands to include and understand their functioning from within himself. But, through harmony with natural law, he does not – or should not – use them.

Frequent mention of the Kundalini is made in esoteric literature and one meets people who claim to have 'awakened' this power. Fortunately for them, this is not normally true, but only the stirrings of subtle energies within them of a less powerful and central nature. Deep mental, emotional and physical purity is required for the safe practice of these forms of yoga. Once enlivened the energy begins to 'rise-up' and any blockages in its path due to impurity of mind can lead to disastrous consequences. Any of the passions can take hold of the practitioner and, with the greater force of enlivened prana behind it, can drive the yogi into greater states of imbalance, inner turmoil and disturbance than that to which even normal people are prone. Even insanity may follow.

Kundalini is sometimes described as being associated with the sacral or sex chakra, because the energy or prana devoted to sex, especially in modern western society, is considerable and represents one of the most difficult of all human energies for the yogi to control and sublimate. Prana, however, has to pass to the Mul chakra for the latter's maintenance and existence and the central nadi reaches down to this centre.

Kundalini is also known as the Serpent Power, because a serpent or snake lies asleep, in coiled form, with the potential to awake and strike with great effect.

An explanation of the pranas as a river is given in Dr. Stone's book: *The Mystic Bible*, 'Which flows out of the etheric (subtle) realm and becomes the gross physical prana, which in turn flows over the nervous system in the body of man. The prana flows over the five tattwas as fields and regions in the human body, as wire-less (subtle) energy, before it becomes the gross prana of nerve impulses and physical action.'

Dr. Stone continues: 'The downward drive for (sexual) sensation wastes the precious pranic energy and binds the senses, the mind, and the soul to this earthward pull. There is little chance for this fine sensory energy to be purified and drawn upward and inward by concentration, when it is exhausted in the downward trend, (towards the base of the physical body). Not only does this waste of energy prevent one from making spiritual progress, but it also robs the rest of the life energy currents necessary for maintaining the physical body in perfect health and vigour. Through this wasting or squandering, it uses more than is naturally apportioned to that centre by the economy of the pattern essence. Only six petals are allotted to this lotus or chakra, out of the total of fifty-two petals on the Tree of Life in the body. The energy goes either up or down. If up, it enriches the mind function and the consciousness and helps to free the soul from bondage.'

The third chakra is the *Manipurak* or *Nabi Chakra*, which is situated near the solar plexus at the umbilicus or navel. The Hindu deities are known as *Vishnu*, the nourisher or sustainer, and *Lakshmi*. This chakra is concerned with physical nourishment and its attribute or guna is that of maintenance or preservation – satvas – which keeps a balance between what physiologists call anabolism and catabolism – the building up and breaking down processes, which taken together are known as metabolism. The western term – the *solar* plexus – is of ancient origin and suggests the heat centre, solar referring to the sun – though many modern interpretations have assumed that 'solar' referred to the radial network of nerves and ganglia, which are supposed to resemble the suns 'rays'. However, the sun is a bright fiery object, emitting light more or less uniformly – not in rays – though the pictorial use of rays has become an established manner of its portrayal.

It is at this centre that we meet with one of the 'skys' experienced from time to time in our inward journey, in the form of the diaphragm. Dr. Stone explains this in *The Mystic Bible*: 'In the human body, the diaphragm is the elastic, functioning firmament which divides (like a valve) the water and earth elements from the fire and air elements.' It is upon this important interaction that life depends. Without diaphragmatic function, there can be no respiration, no heart-beat, no proper elimination nor assimilation, nor motion. It is a fixed stabilizer of bodily function.'

This chakra has eight petals or letters, its colour is dark red and the tattwa or element controlling it is Agni – fire, the material field of which is the condition of heat. Fire is purifying and dissolving like water, but carries the process much further. It also raises the vibrations of all substances touched by it, thus preparing them for the next higher stage – air or the gaseous state. There is no generation nor preservation of life without heat in some degree.

It is the fiery, warming and nourishing characteristics of the energy disseminated through this chakra that is responsible for metabolism. Its endocrine counterpart is the pancreas which controls not only the fiery, digestive processes, but also, through insulin, the sugar metabolism and balance of the bodily caloric or heat-production biochemistry.

It is clear, of course, that this kind of description runs in a different mode to that of conventional, western scientific or medical thinking. This is because we are dealing here with a vertical spectrum of energies, out of which the lower energies and matter are created. Modern scientific method deals with horizontal relationships and interaction at the lowest levels of this spectrum, seeking to find the 'ultimate' energy fields or particles, not realizing that the source of gross material manifestation is beyond the area of activity of outward instrumentation.

The fourth centre or plexus is the *Hriday* or *Heart Chakra*. It controls the body circulation, blood and respiration. Its functions are protection, destruction, and dissolution of the physical body, so its guna is tamas. It is situated at the cardiac or heart plexus and its Hindu deities are *Shiva* and *Parvathi*. Its tattwa is air or the gaseous state – Vayu. It has twelve petals or letters and its colour is green.

Dr. Stone again says in *The Mystic Bible*: 'Here, we also find the mystic chalice spoken of as a cup; namely the heart, the mixing bowl of the life principle (prana) with the air, fire, and water elements. Prana or the universal life force uses oxygen as a conveyor and we breathe it in as air. The Bible clearly states that the 'life is in the blood'. If the chemical oxygen was the life principle itself, we could prolong life indefinitely under an oxygen tent, which is not the case'.

The heart centre is thus a protector and distributor of energies, this function being mirrored in the newly discovered role of the thymus gland. This gland, considered until recently to be an evolutionary vestige of no importance, is now known to be the master orchestrator of the bodily immune system through a number of similar hormones, known collectively as thymosin. The body's immune system is the biochemical and physiological mechanism by which it protects itself from outside 'invaders' – either chemical, bacteriological or viral – as well as internal toxins and biochemical 'errors' and 'upsets'.

Greed, or overprotection of one's rights under natural law, is the human weakness and energy imbalance of this chakra at the emotional level. Those who have risen in consciousness above the grosser influences of intense attachment, lust and anger are often given to heart problems as they struggle to work in the world with their increased sensitivity, through the more synthesizing and collective or group aspects of this centre.

The fifth centre is the *Kanth*, *Vishudhi* or *Throat Chakra* which lies near the cervical plexus or throat. The Hindu deity is *Shakti*, the mother-goddess or source of power of the deities below. It has sixteen petals or letters and its colour is blue. It is the seat of the etheric tattwa or akash which sustains the three lower chakras of water, fire and air and their corresponding gunas of creation, preservation and destruction. Without akash, the intellect (buddhi) of man cannot manifest itself. That is, man's capacity for rational thought requires the presence of the energy field of akash.

While the Hindus talk of Shakti as the mother-goddess or energy source for the lower centres, in western terms this is reflected in the thyroid and parathyroid endocrine glands which perform a regulatory and controlling function upon all body metabolism.

In particular, the throat centre governs the vocal as well as the pulmonary and bronchial organs. Emotional shock therefore can bring on spasm and constriction of the bronchial system resulting in sobbing, sighs and even attacks of asthma.

Akash being the element or material state associated with this chakra as well as with human rationality, the strength and weakness associated with this chakra is that of truthfulness and honesty and their reverse. The 'fast-talker' working from his lower emotional centres will have a tendency to incorrectness in his (or her) expression of events and feelings – both outwardly and from within themselves, while the one who operates from the next higher, eye centre, or further in, stands a better chance of expressing themselves with honesty.

True honesty, requiring an absence of ego – since ego is in itself an illusion or dishonest representation of our reality – is one of the most difficult of virtues to imbibe. Indeed, it will never come by a search for honesty itself, but as a bi-product of the inner search for the higher Truth or Reality deep within all of us.

The last major centre within the subtle physical body, and the only one with which truely spiritual practices are concerned, is the *Ajna Chakra* or *Do-Dal-Kanwal* – the two petalled lotus, on a level with the base of the physical eyes, one petal of which is white and the other black. This is the headquarters of our soul and mind during the waking state. From this point, the currents of our soul have come down and spread throughout our whole body – into every cell and hair. The presiding deity therefore is Atma – a combination of man's soul and mind. All centres below this are under its control and all deities in them are therefore *subordinate* to the control of his mind and spirit. All these six chakras are therefore within the realm of the physical universe or Pinda.

Thus we find that the pituitary gland with its two lobes, reflections, perhaps, of the two petals of the ajna chakra, plays a major orchestrating role over the lower endocrine glands, with linkages to higher centres in the brain itself. The pituitary operates within a finely tuned feedback loop, regulating the activity of all the other lower endocrine glands, just as the ajna chakra regulates and is linked to the energy flow of the lower chakras. Molecules, after all, hormonal or otherwise, are really only a vibration of energy, of atomic and sub-atomic forces and particles. We have a good deal more to say on these energy relationships as we progress through this book.

The posterior pituitary lobe is really a separate gland,

whose hormones are manufactured in the hypothalamus. In fact, it is probable that the two petals of the ajna chakra are more correctly related to the anterior pituitary on the one hand and the hypothalamus/posterior pituitary, on the other. There is considerable hormonal interplay between the functioning of the hypothalamus and the anterior lobe of the pituitary. Indeed, the entire chakra, element and neuroendocrine system is a fascinating subject and one which I hope to explore in a future book.

The ajna centre also provides the subtle energy fields required for the operation of the main sense organs and their linkage to brain functions – all the major sense organs being located in the head.

Ego and self-consciousness are perhaps the inherent weakness of this centre, though in reality the seat of human ego lies in a yet higher centre, as we describe below. All other human weaknesses have their source in ego, in a sense of self. Without ego, there can be no lust, anger, greed, attachment, dishonesty or any of the other subdivisions of these energy imbalances of our mental-emotional complex, that make us all so human.

It must be clearly understood that *these six centres in subtle matter do not contain spirituality* but only material forces. For real spirituality we have to ascend above the eyes, into the next division of creation which we can do, directly, from where we are at present, from behind the two eyes.

Many occult schools talk of a seventh, crown chakra. This relates to a bundling together of the astral and causal chakras which lie above the physical chakras. Thus the thousand petalled lotus of the astral region is sometimes referred to as the crown chakra. What is important is that one understands that those energies are above the physical body and subtle physical energies. To really understand what any of these energies are like, there is no substitute for inner experience, to go there and see for yourself.

The *Eye Centre* or Do-Dal-Kanwal is as far as concentration and meditation on the six chakras can take the soul. The progress of those who follow *Pranayama* (the practice of rhythmic breathing) stops at this centre, where these nadis and the pranas merge in *Chitakash* (the sky of the body within) the place of their origin. They cannot go beyond this stage, for no power or energy current can carry one further than its origin. From here some souls realize their plight and take the help of the *Three Canals* or streams and manage to reach their origin, which is Sahans-dal-Kanwal, the thousand petalled lotus. Having described these regions or chakras, we should thoroughly understand that they are explanations not of the physical effect, as we might see it operating in the observable anatomy of man's physical functioning. They are the subtle energy pattern governing these functions, in the subtle part of the physical body. It is as though one could see the 'cause' of which the physical functioning is the 'effect'. However, one whose higher spiritual consciousness is awakened can see the workings of these energies from within themselves, with an inner eye of perception. It can only have been in this way, and from such souls, that the meridians of acupuncture, for example, were mapped and made available as a science. Even now, we meet people quite frequently, who are aware to one degree or another of the flow of subtle physical energies. This intuitive faculty develops with practice in some of those working in these fields of healing or as a by-product of meditation. I have met a number of people who have this gift.

Just above the two-petalled lotus is another centre known as *Char-Dal-Kanwal* or four petalled lotus, whose function is to supply the four-fold *Antashkarans* with centres of action. The antashkarans are the four faculties which give us our physical mind and which provide the energy fields in which our thoughts are manifested. The old adage: 'Thoughts are things', becomes apparent to direct observation at this level. The four faculties are: *Manas*, *Buddhi*, *Chit*, and *Ahankar*. Each of the petals of this lotus has its own sound and these four complete the fifty-two letters of the Sanskrit alphabet. This is the lowest of the six centres of Anda (astral region) and lies nearest to Pinda (physical region).

Buddhi is the faculty of discrimination and of intellect, of impersonal consciousness of the Jiva, or soul imprisoned in the human body. It makes decisions based upon the impressions gained from the chit and manas. Whilst buddhi is the discriminatory faculty, it has in itself no power to initiate action, being impersonal. Buddhi is the detached, objective logic behind intellectual functioning. It is the power of rationality, though infused with understanding of morality and the higher qualities of life according to the degree of consciousness of the individual and his contact with the higher or inner energies of his own being.

Buddhi, however, requires a degree of personalization in order for it to find expression as an individual human being. This is the faculty of *Ahankar*, of personal awareness. It is ahankar which identifies with the perceptions of the senses and the subsequent responses. Buddhi and ahankar together make up the 'experiencer'. Ahankar is thus the executive faculty, implementing the decisions, impressions, habit-patterns and so on, passed to it by the other three faculties. It is the I-ness of the individual, whereby he differentiates himself from all else and distinguishes his own interests from those of others. When out of balance, as it is with most of us, it becomes human ego, the source of all human weakness.

Manas is mind-stuff, per se. It is that which registers impressions from the senses and its reactions are instantaneous according to its habits or grooves of previous experience. The faculty of enjoyment and of desire is couched in manas. The experiencer is affected by the material world in five separate ways, giving rise in him to the sensations of sound and hearing, colour and form and sight, touch and feel, taste, and smell. Manas thus receives sensory impressions from the 'outside', but it is itself quite automatic and requires the existence of buddhi and ahankar to give it life and for its activities to be experienced. Buddhi surveys the impressions gained by manas and makes intelligent selection and decisions thereon, whilst ahankar becomes the executive, personal faculty when any action is to be taken.

While manas is the immediate and present faculty of cognition, the last faculty of the fourfold human mind is that of *Chit*. Chit[1] is memory. It is the storehouse of all the impressions gained by manas. Psychologists talk of short-term and long-term memory. If manas is short-term memory, then chit is the mental substance in which long-

---

[1] As with many Sanskrit terms, the word *Chit* is used in other contexts where it means something different. Thus many yoga practitioners are aware of the phrase, *Sat, Chit, Anand* as attributes of the soul, translated as Truth, Consciousness and Bliss. *Chit* here, clearly has a somewhat different meaning.

term impressions are lodged. Thus, ahankar and buddhi draw automatically on this reservoir when making their decisions and actions.

Summary

The Great Master, Maharaj Sawan Singh Ji, once wrote in a letter to a western disciple many years ago: 'Sach Khand (Sat Purush) and the stages above it constitute the pure Spiritual Region. This is the only unchangeable part. Brahmanda (causal region), Anda (astral region) and Pinda (physical region) are changeable, and therefore perishable. Leaving the pure Spiritual Region aside, the remaining parts – Brahmanda, Anda and Pinda – are related to one another as the image is related to the object. Anda is the reflection of Brahmanda, and Pinda is the reflection of Anda, just as the sun and its reflection in water and the reflection on a wall from the surface are related to one another. The sun is above in the sky with all its magnificence and power. The image in the water has the appearance of the sun but has lost much of its magnificence. The reflection on the wall is only a hazy patch of light, distorted and devoid of glory. Pinda is a copy of Anda, and Anda is a copy of Brahmanda. The so-called man is thus a copy of the copy, leaving aside the Pure Spirit. 'Just to give you an idea how the corresponding centres in Pinda, Anda, and Brahmanda ressemble one another, like the sun and its images; the lowest centre in Pinda is at the rectum, with red colour and four petals. The corresponding centre in Anda is the lowest centre, just above the eyes, with red colour and four petals. The corresponding centre in Brahmanda is Trikuti, with red colour and four petals. The red sun of Trikuti is reflected in the four petalled lotus of the antashkarans, just above the eyes, and this in turn is reflected down at the rectum as the dull red-coloured four-petalled lotus.

'The majority of systems of concentration start from the rectum and then slowly work up the attention to the eye focus. Some start from the heart centre and then slowly work up to the eye centre; for in the case of ordinary men, the headquarters of the attention is not the eyes but the heart (the emotional centre). Man rises to the eye centre only when thinking deeply, and again sinks down below the eyes. Dream and sleep states are caused by the attention sinking below the eye focus.

'The system of the saints starts with concentration from the eye focus. They do not concentrate at any centre below the eyes. The argument is simple. Man is normally working from the heart centre. So man is sitting at the middle of the mountain whose base is the rectum and the top is the eye and the heart is the midway point. Going down to the rectum and then coming up is a waste of time and energy. So saints straightway put the eye focus as the first goal to reach the top. There is a natural capacity in man to rise up to the eyes, although he does not stick to it. This last fact is the only drawback. Saints therefore remove the drawback by repeatedly going up to the eye focus; and the eye focus by practice becomes the headquarters of attention. Changing the headquarters of attention upwards is going towards the light, step by step.

'Power lies in concentration, no matter at what centre it is concentrated. However, the higher the centre, the greater the power, and the greater the peace. Entering and sticking to any centre in Pinda, or parts below the eyes is the study of the reflection of a reflection. Saints have discarded entering into Pinda. They sit at the eye focus, withdraw the current up to this centre and start off to Anda and Brahmanda.'

A present living Master, Maharaj Charan Singh Ji clarifies the general approach when he advises (in the book *The Master Answers*): 'We should not get confused with how many regions or stages have been described (by the mystics). Actually, it is the same journey and they are not watertight compartments. The journey has to be described in one way or another; so this language just describes it. Some have described it as just two regions; some have classified the two regions into four, some five, and some into eight. Actually it is the same journey, and covers the same territory, which is classified as consisting of two, four, five, or eight (regions).'

Mysticsm, Subtle Energy and Human Experience

Intellect, Intuition and Psychic Phenomena

The complexity of the energy currents in the subtle physical body is immense, surpassed only by the multiplicity of forms, actions and reactions of the gross physical plane itself. Unravelling the interactions of biochemical, physiological, sub-atomic and molecular physical processes is enough to keep a conventional scientific community busy for centuries. The real solution to the understanding of these processes lies in the understanding of the energy blueprints that control, regulate and create them. This process, however, is best understood by viewing from within, by inner concentration, rather than by intellectual analysis.

Indeed, when viewed from below, from the human standpoint, and using only intellect and intuition as tools for our understanding, the complex picture can never be unravelled. The possible inter-reactions are practically infinite in their manifestation. Intellect itself is only another one of the multitudinous energies of the universe. It is Buddhi, one of the antashkarans, the attributes of mind, only a reflection of a ray from the Universal Mind, a part of the lowest chakra in the astral universe.

The physical mind – the antashkarans – has its purpose: that of regulating life on this plane and providing enough understanding of it to function (more or less!) successfully, but the physical mind can never provide a full cosmic understanding along with complete knowledge of the Ultimate Cause. It is in itself only another part of the cosmos that requires understanding.

One can never really understand a thing by standing apart from it. To know a thing, one must become that thing, to allow it to be a part of oneself, to merge with it, to let it become a part of one's consciousness. Intellectual analysis, however positively applied, is essentially a tool of duality, leading easily to separateness and personal egotism. Characteristically, the intellectual person feels himself superior to his 'lesser-endowed' fellow humans, however hard he may struggle against it. And yet the intellect is only one aspect of a human being. Other human qualities of affection, generosity, tolerance, co-operation and understanding are really of more value than intellectual capability. And these can be found in great abundance in illiterate people as readily as in the educated. Some would say more so. So to understand, in the highest sense, one has to *become* the object of which understanding is required. How does this come about?

Remember that man is the microcosm, the entire mystic energy dance is reflected within him. By means of the correct practice of meditation, a soul can rise up by concentration upon the inner energy currents. There are many forms of yoga and meditation, following different energy currents to their particular source. The highest form of meditation, then, is that which follows the course of the Life Stream, the Shabd, the primal creative outpouring, back to its Source. This is also the most difficult practice since the obstacles in the shape of the multitudinous downwardly directed currents are the most severe.

As a soul rises up, the nature and structure of creation through the energy patterns and vibrations below, become to him, an open book. They become a part of his consciousness and not only does he have full knowledge of them, but he also has full control over them, should he wish to exercise it. Thus it is possible to perform miracles.

To a dog or a cat, the creation of an electric fire is a miracle. They have not the consciousness to understand the mechanisms of its creation. Man, with his superior amount of the akash element, can understand its processes enough to be able to build such a fire, though full knowledge of the structure of matter and the sub-atomic energy reactions and transformations is not required for its manufacture.

Similarly, as a soul goes within, wherever the energy pathways are contained within his consciousness, he can, at will, manipulate these pathways and create apparent miracles. Miracles, however, require energy from within and disciples of true spiritual disciplines where such powers are likely to become manifest in them are strictly enjoined not to waste their energy performing 'party tricks', but to preserve their energy for further inward advancement.

All individuals have different energy constitutions. The basic patterns are the same, but we are all manifestly different from each other. There are those who have a development within their subtle physical energies – the chakras, the pranas, the akash, the antashkarans – in excess of the average. These people we call psychics, clairvoyants, healers and so on. In the majority of such cases, the individuals themselves have little or no control over their faculty. It comes and goes. Those of them who have practised a specific form of spiritual discipline will have a greater control, though through that control such people may cease to use their abilities in an outward way.

All the energy of such ESP (extra sensory perception) or psi phenomena as metal-bending, psychokinesis, mental telepathy and so on, lies in the subtle energy area between the gross physical and the antashkarans. The application of mental concentration in such gifted people, opens up the energy pathways from the physical mind through to the object of concentration and the phenomenon takes place.

The energy of our destiny or karma for this life is recorded in the antashkarans. It is from here that our outward life as well as our personality has its roots. Personality is also a part of destiny – part of the outworking of the energy of karma that makes us do what we have to do. Our personality partially determines the decisions we make – and this is according to our destiny. Access to this information, this energy of destiny karma, and hence of the future, is thus available and so we have clairvoyants. Such people, however, are human, like the rest of us and can make mistakes in the interpretation of the intuitions they receive. Or even, with their best intentions, their own desires and imagination can lead them astray either in the foretelling of their own destiny or that of others. This happens as much in the daily life of everyone, as in such gifted people.

In fact, we are all affected by the subtle energies of the physical universe. It is simply that sometimes we are more aware or conscious of it than at others. At this time in our human history, the numbers of people who are aware of the subtle energy vibrations and who have intuitions and knowledge of inner things is increasing. Just like a wave which breaks simultaneously, but independently, at different points along its length, so too is there a generation of people in all parts of the world who are simultaneously experiencing an awakening within their own consciousness.

Astrologers call this the beginnings of the Aquarian Age, the New Age. It began around the turn of the century with such groups as the Theosophists and Rudolf Steiner. It moved slowly, but was quickened by the negative polarity of the two world wars. It began an acceleration in the fifties, gained young blood and new strength in the sixties, began to mature in the seventies and is taking on deep practical shape in the nineteen eighties.

But this knowledge always existed in the East. Indeed, even now, despite the unrest and westernization, there are still places where the atmosphere seems permeated with the ages of spirituality. In the West, it is only here and there that historically one finds traces of true mysticism.

Just as with the inner ascent to higher regions, there are valves which permit easy downward flow of energy and spirit, but are difficult in ascent and require a tremendous degree of concentration, before passing through into an area of expansion and calm, so too can the extreme polarities of positive and negative, present in current world conditions be interpreted as a whirling of the energy required to break through into an area and age of greater peace and harmony.

Never before in recorded history has man had the ability to destroy himself and his planet so completely and utterly. And never before has there been such easy access to and such widespread understanding of spiritual and mystic realities. I am frequently surprised that people who one might have suspected would react with scepticism to such thoughts as are expressed here, in fact exhibit a degree of open-mindedness that does credit to our human race!

I do not say that a healthy discrimination and mental appraisal of facts is not good. Quite the reverse. But the dismissal out of hand, on a mostly emotional rather than rational level, is an attitude adopted less and less frequently than even just a decade ago. It is part of a continuum, a process: in past ages, heads would have rolled if such thoughts and ideas were made public. The history of the persecution of saintly or simply harmless people is a definite blot on the landscape of human behaviour. This is not to say that such intolerance is now obliterated. That is unfortunately untrue. It is simply that there is a general mood abroad that as long as someone or some group is harmless, then let them be, perhaps even investigated, to see what they have to offer in terms of human advancement.

Mystic Knowledge

Mystics rarely speak of their inner experiences because they understand the incredulity with which their descriptions would be met. Here and there, however, we do find descriptions with remarkably similar aspects, found in all cultures and from all ages. Dr. Johnson has collected together some of these in his: *Path of the Masters* from the Christian anthology: *Mystic Experiences of Medieval Saints* and I present a few of them here. To what height on the mystic ladder these mystics had advanced is impossible to tell, nor is it of anything other than academic importance, but the similarity and validity of their experiences is unquestionable.

'After this prayer, I once found myself inundated with a vivid light; it seemed to me that a veil was lifted up from before my eyes of the spirit, and all the truths of human science, even those that I had not studied, became manifest to me by an infused knowledge. This state of intuition lasted for about twenty-four hours, and then, as if the veil had fallen again, I found myself as ignorant as before.'

St. Francis Xavier

'As he was ... sitting on the banks of the Gardenera his mind was suddenly filled with a new and strange illumination, so that in one moment, and without any sensible image, or appearance, certain things pertaining to the mysteries of the faith, together with other truths of natural science, were revealed to him, and this so abundantly and so clearly, that he himself said that if all the spiritual light which his spirit had received from God up to the time when he was more than sixty years old, could be collected into one, it seemed to him that all of this knowledge could not equal what was at that moment conveyed to his soul.'

St. Ignatius

'And as he stood there praying, he was suddenly raised above himself in such a wonderful manner, that he could not afterwards account for it, and the Lord revealed to him the whole beauty and glory of the firmament and of every created thing so that his longing was fully satisfied. But afterwards, when he came to himself, the prior could get nothing out of him than that he had received such an unspeakable rapture from his perfect knowledge of creation, that it was beyond human understanding'

Herman Joseph

'He saw a light which banished away the darkness of the night – upon this sight a marvelous strange thing followed. The whole world gathered, as it were, under one beam of the sun, was presented before his eyes. For by that super-natural light, the capacity of the inward soul is enlarged. But albeit the world was gathered together before his eyes, yet were not the heaven and earth drawn into any lesser form than they be of themselves, but the soul or the beholder was more enlarged.'

St. Benedict

'When our Lord suspends the understanding and makes it cease from its actions – (by this she means that the normal activity of the mind is brought to a stand-still, made motionless) – He puts before it that which astonishes it and occupies it; so that without making any reflections (without reasoning things out) it shall comprehend in a moment more than we could comprehend in many years, with all the efforts in the world.'

St. Theresa

The physicist and author, Fritjof Capra describes a similar experience in the preface to his book: *The Tao of Physics*. He writes: 'Five years ago, I had a beautiful experience which set me on the road to the writing of this book. I was sitting by the ocean one late summer afternoon, watching the waves rolling in and feeling the rhythm of my breathing, when I suddenly became aware of my whole environment as being engaged in a gigantic cosmic dance. ... As I sat on that beach my former experiences (his intellectual knowledge of physics) came to 'life'; I 'saw' cascades of energy coming down from outer space, in which particles were created and destroyed in rhythmic pulses; I 'saw' the atoms of the elements and those of my body participating in this cosmic dance of energy; I felt its rhythm and I 'heard' its sound, and at that moment I *knew* that this was the Dance of Shiva, the Lord of Dancers, worshipped by the Hindus.'

Finally, let me quote from Paramhansa Yogananda's well-known and much-loved book: *Autobiography of a Yogi*. One day, Yogananda's Guru, taking pity on his beloved disciple's struggles with meditation gave him a spontaneous experience of cosmic consciousness. He writes: 'My body became immovably rooted; breath was drawn out of my lungs as if by some huge magnet. Soul and mind instantly lost their physical bondage, and streamed out like a fluid piercing light from every pore. The flesh was as though dead, yet in my intense awareness I knew that I had never before been fully alive. My sense of identity was no longer narrowly confined to a body, but embraced the circumambient atoms. People on distant streets seemed to be moving gently over my remote periphery. The roots of plants and trees appeared through a dim transparency of the soil; I discerned the inward flow of their sap.

'The whole vicinity lay bare before me. My ordinary frontal vision was now changed to a vast spherical sight, simultaneously all-perceptive. Through the back of my head I saw men strolling far down Rai Ghat Lane, and noticed also a white cow who was leisurely approaching. When she reached the space in front of the open ashram gate, I observed her as though with my physical eyes. As she passed by, behind the brick wall, I saw her still.

'All objects within my panoramic gaze trembled and vibrated like quick motion pictures. My body, Master's, the pillared courtyard, the furniture and floor, the trees and sunshine, occasionally became violently agitated, until all melted into a luminescent sea; even as sugar crystals, thrown into a glass of water, dissolve after being shaken. The unifying light alternated with materialization of forms, the metamorphoses revealing the law of cause and effect (karma) in creation.

'An oceanic joy broke upon the calm endless shores of my soul. The Spirit of God, I realized, is exhaustless Bliss; His body is countless tissues of light. A swelling glory within me began to envelop towns, continents, the earth, solar and stellar systems, tenuous nebulae, and floating universes. The entire cosmos, gently luminous, like a city seen afar at night, glimmered within the infinitude of my being. The dazzling light beyond the sharply edged global outlines faded somewhat at the farthest edges; there I could see a mellow radiance, ever-undiminished. It was indescribably subtle; the planetary pictures were formed of a grosser light.

'The divine dispersion of rays poured from an Eternal Source, blazing into galaxies, transfigured with ineffable auras. Again and again I saw the creative beams condense into constellations, then resolve into sheets of transparent flame. By rhythmic reversions, sextillion worlds passed into diaphanous lustre, then fire became firmament.

'I cognized the centre of the empyrean as a point of intuitive perception in my heart. Irradiating splendour issued from my nucleus to every part of the universal structure. Blissful *amrita*, the nectar of immortality, pulsed through me with a quicksilverlike fluidity. The creative voice of God I heard resounding as *Aum*, the vibration of the Cosmic Motor.'

There is really nothing one can add to these descriptions – they speak for themselves. Experience is the reality, these words are just a shadow.

Cosmic Philosophy, Mysticism and Modern Science

Many of the apparent paradoxes and conflicting points of view in all aspects of human thought – religious, philosophical, ideological or scientific – are dissolved when considered in the light of a true cosmic philosophy. Although, as we have said previously, true understanding can only be attained by going within and studying the energy pathways from inside, intellectual endeavour has a use and validity, but only within the confines for which, in the cosmic order, it is intended. Just as one does not expect to see with one's knees, so too we should not expect the intellect to be capable of truly understanding energies higher than itself!

The problem is, of course, that our subtle constitution is not at all clear to us. Many feel that they are their body and that when the body dies, they die. Some feel that they are their mind, but that the mind is only the 'self-conscious' aspect of the physical body, which therefore dies with the body. Others, who have a strong inner awareness of their own self, realize that they are not the body and that there is some more real part of themselves which survives the physical death of the body, but what it is, they have no philosophy in which to express it. Others have a religious or philosophical framework into which such questions are channelled which prevent the individual from asking himself the basic questions of 'What am I?' and 'What is happening here?' Moreover, everyone is absorbed to a greater or lesser degree, with the events of the day, which attract the senses and confuse the mind with their requirements for attention, making it an easy matter to neglect the all important cosmic and mystic questions, even to ridicule them.

Hence, the intellect is confused by emotion and its own limited rationality, and runs along its own course, largely undirected from within, controlling the individual, rather than being used consciously as a valuable instrument, but with certain limitations. It speaks a loud 'I' within the mind and with that comes an identity and ego which it is hard to relinquish and which reacts vehemently when challenged with ideas to which it is not accustomed.

The intellect works by analysis and comparison. Paradoxes arise from its limitations. It is just like the children's story of the ten blind men asked to describe an elephant: each man caught hold of a different part of the beast and described it differently. To one it was like a tall pillar; to another it was large, floppy and thin; to another it was long, thick, round and flexible. In discussing their different experiences they got into an argument which was unresolvable until, perhaps, they realized that they were all correct.

Each one was describing his own experience as if it were universal, rather than limited.

Similarly, with paradoxes, all the aspects can all be true – there are many facets to a diamond which give rise to conflicting descriptions. Intellectually intense people need to be more 'laid-back'. An over identification of self with an idea makes a person threatened when the idea is called into question. In past ages and even in some parts of the world today, a fanatical identification with a certain way of thinking leads such people to find excuses for murdering or imprisoning those of other philosophies. One name for it is prejudice – and its roots go deep into the human mind.

One of the beauties of mystic or cosmic philosophy is that it has some sort of an answer to all questions and a place for all philosophies and modes of thought. There is nothing which is outside its scope and yet, at all stages it says: 'This thinking is only an indication, only a pointer or incentive. If you want real knowledge, you have to find it within yourself. And these are the steps you have to follow.'

Modern physics, since it addresses itself directly to sub-atomic energy relationships is probably at the leading edge of human, intellectual analysis of physical energy patterns. In fact, there are many parallels in thinking between modern physics and mystic philosophy. Fritjof Capra in his book: *The Tao of Physics* provides us with an excellent study and survey of these parallels of meaning and nomenclature or jargon.

Mystic philosophy and modern physics both say that there is nothing but energy patterns, pathways and relationships. Even classical thermodynamics recognizes that we are in a closed energy system, that in nature you cannot get something for nothing. Modern physics, in tracing that 'something' goes deeper into matter discovering that what appears as solid to us is no more than a cosmic energy dance, that in macroscopic analogy sometimes bears resemblances to particles, sometimes to waves and fields.

Some modern theorists talk of 'ghost matter'. For any particle to exist, they say, there must be an energy vibration, a blueprint of it in an energy field which we cannot as yet identify. This they call 'ghost matter' – ghost electrons and protons etc, or virtual matter – something which comes before the existence of physical matter.

This is subtle matter, subtle energy, as understood by mystic philosophy and described previously. And as we saw, energy is projected downwards, 'created' from above or within.

CHAPTER 3

Spiritual, Mental and Physical Energies

The discussion of the previous chapters now puts us in a position to understand healing and disease in its truest sense.

The surge of interest in the West during the last five years in alternative medicine or natural means of healing is a practical crystallization of the mental and spiritual awakening of the generation who reached maturity during the late sixties and seventies. Many of the therapies were already present, others have come into being only recently or have been imported, sometimes with modifications from older and wiser cultures.

All sufferings and relative happinesses are due to our separation from the One Source of all. Harmony, rhythm and vitality in the energy patterns which surround the soul result in health, well-being and prosperity. Disharmony, inertia and negativity project as ill-health and disease. No soul, after descending into the mind region will ever be surrounded by totally positive influences. In the regions of duality, positive and negative are fundamental attributes at whatever level we examine creation.

In the physical body, we find a combination of positive and negative tendencies. If the body were all positive, if the sub-atomic and subtle energies were purely of creative and positive vibration, then the body would never die, never suffer ill-health. Moreover, no cells would ever die and be replaced. The body would simply get fatter and fatter! If the body were composed of all negative aspects, it could never come into existence. It would wither away rapidly in sickness, disease and death.

Healing can be considered at all levels. The true healing is one that removes the root cause of ill-health. Therefore, the only true cure is one that takes us back to our Source. At levels other than this, healing is temporary and relative. It has a place, and an important one, but is not permanent.

We are like prisoners in a jailhouse. When a philanthropist comes and makes social reforms to improve our lot, it is valuable. Better food, warm clothes and more pleasant surroundings provide nourishment for our being. But one who comes with a key that lets us escape from the prison puts the work of the philanthropist into its proper proportions. Such is the nature of all philanthropic healing – welcome, but relative.

The Healing of a True Mystic

The one who heals by taking us out of the jailhouse, away from the wheel of birth and death, is a Mystic, a Satguru or Saint. He heals only those whom he takes under his protection, in his own lifetime. There will have been previous mystics for those who came before and will be others for those who come after. Healing requires the individual touch of being to being. A true mystic, of the highest order, takes the soul into his care. He takes into his own arms the administration of the entanglements of energy patterns and relationships, the causes and effects, the karmas with which the soul has surrounded itself during its multitude of births and its stay in the worlds of the physical, astral and causal realms.

A ball of string cannot disentangle itself, a thin cloth cannot extract itself from a thorny bush, a man cannot escape unaided from a quicksand. Every action made of itself results in further entanglement. The need of the Mystic Healer is primary.

Spiritual Healing.

Within the sub-astral realms of the Universal Mind, there are souls, often of good intention, love and humility, who perform what is known as spiritual healing, for the souls living on the physical plane. Some are living in a physical body, others are in higher regions – mostly sub-astral, working through a medium in the physical world. Their mechanism is to consciously or unconsciously take onto themselves some of the negative tendencies and entanglements or karmas of those they desire to heal. This is good for the one who is healed, but the healer always does it at his own cost. He has to take the negativity onto himself. Healing from this level, therefore, however pure the motive, is not recommended by mystics of the highest order. Rather, they specifically advise against it.

The same applies to yogis and mystics who have not gone beyond the realm of the Universal Mind and who take on some of the karmas of their disciples. It is done, ultimately, at the cost of their own spirituality. Their 'eternity' being a relative one, the reservoir of their spiritual strength is ultimately exhausted, because it is not consciously linked to the everlasting source of spirituality.

In fact, the word spiritual, in the context of this kind of healing is, strictly speaking, incorrect. It is a healing of mental, emotional and physical energies, using mental and very occasionally higher mental, astral or causal power. The spirit does not come into it. True spiritual healing is to free the spirit or soul from the mind, and that can only be performed by a true mystic. The spirit is then healed of its connection with mind and matter. In fact, the word 'astral' is very loosely used by the majority of western people. These days very few people reach the astral and at this level the pull begins to be upwards. There is no encouragement for it to travel downwards to cure physically.

I am aware that many good and loving people are involved in this kind of work and that benefits are felt by those who are healed. But it is indeed a trap of the mind for such kind-hearted and evolved humans and the burden of the karmas of those healed often leads such healers to distress in later life. Many of them both look and feel burdened beyond the average. There is no need for us to become a carrier of other's burdens, we have enough karmas of our own. There are many ways of healing that do not drain one's own energies.

Positive Thinking, Visualization, Psychological Therapies

Following down the energy pathways, we come once again to the antashkarans, the physical mind, the energy centre in which we experience thought. The healing given by true mystics takes place from the highest source and constitutes a complete cure. Spiritual healing comes from within the sub-astral, the astral and occasionally the causal regions. All other forms of healing known to us come from energies between the level of the antashkarans down to the gross physical.

The thinking processes of humans, the complex energy patterns within the antashkarans, project downwards and along with the multitudinous energy currents from above, through the chakras and the pranas and other subtle energies, these all precipitate finally as the physical body.

Thus it is that all psychosomatic effects take place. When people say: 'It is just psychological', they normally mean that it can be dismissed as something unreal. But this is not so. It is very real. It is energy. There has to be an energy pathway connecting the cause with the effect. The cause is the thought, the effect is the disharmony, disease or psychosomatic result in the physical body. If something is 'psychological' it is serious. In fact, all disease has a psychological aspect. We are one complex energy system, not a collection of separate systems. All aspects of energy are then manifested at all levels within our physical being – physical, subtle, emotional and mental.

The proponents of positive thinking, therefore, are absolutely correct. Not only do positive thoughts reflect in the body as better health, but through the same energy pathways, they reflect outwardly in the manifestation of energy patterns in our environment and activities.

You may have noticed, for example, how some people can make things work for them and others are a disaster area! It is not simply that the one has a better 'gift' with his hands in a purely mechanical sense. Having worked for over fifteen years in the computer world at the University of Cambridge, I noticed many times how certain engineers only had to appear on the scene for the equipment to start working once again. Also, the equipment would go wrong more frequently with certain operators than others or conversely, everything would run smoothly until certains operators went on vacation. The subtle energy force field around each of us effects the electrical qualities of sensitive electronic components. A person with harmonious, balanced vibrations will get more life out of components than one with a jarring, unbalanced atmosphere about them.

As a manufacturer and retailer supplying thousands of goods over a wide spectrum of products, I have also noticed how certain individuals or companies consistently have problems. With so many thousands of customers, there is bound to be the odd faulty product, which one is always ready to remedy. But it is way beyond the bounds of coincidence that certain customers will time and again draw the problems to themselves. The product can get lost in the post, it is the one in a thousand that is faulty, a part is missing, a page is printed upside down in a book or is missing, the product keeps on failing, the replacement sent goes wrong, we send incorrect goods and so on. Things that happen once in several thousand all fall on the one person! There are people who are always lucky – they are always in the right place at the right time. They just catch the train, they buy something just in time to beat a price increase, paint falls from decorators up a ladder and just misses them, they normally have an easy positive attitude. Things flow easily for them. They are nature's 'survivors'.

Others just miss trains, always pay more than they need, get hit by falling bricks and have a pretty negative approach to life! They are nature's 'victims'.

Mental attitude affects the harmony in the subtle energies, it affects the vibrations of a person, and it all happens from there.

Similarly, with Gestalt and various kinds of psychotherapy designed to open up the free flow of energy from within to the outside. The problem with such therapies is that they become self-perpetuating, a strong habit or groove in the energy of the antashkarans. The person is helped, within this sphere, but their attention becomes so focused on this level of being, that they find it difficult to move on from this manner of expression.

There is, therefore, a balance. We talk to ourselves, try to influence ourselves in good directions, get good advice from friends or even various kinds of therapist when occasion demands, but for those who seek to go higher, it is best not to get too involved at this level.

Just as it is impossible ever to sort out and identify all the inter-relationships of physical things by mental analysis or physical observation, so too is it impossible to identify and characterize the elements of energy that make up the personality. Moreover, it excites the tendency to think: 'I', to enlarge our sense of ego. It depends too, as always, on the individual. Some folk are in more of a psychological tangle than others and may need specific therapeutic help. With others, a healthy degree of non-self-indulgent intro-spection, which comes naturally with spiritual practices and meditation, is all that is required. We do not need to get 'heavy', we can be light and have simple, loving fun!

Just as an example of self-healing and what can be achieved through the power of one's own mind, let me quote from the author and friend of mine, George Sand-with, who spent many years in Africa as a surveyor and also in the army during the second world war. He tells the story of how their convoy was ambushed by Gurage tribesman shortly after the Italian occupation of Ethiopia in 1941.

'Firing furiously from the windows of our truck, we stopped to pick up a wounded Gurage, throwing him in the back... After escaping from the ambush, we examined our Gurage. A bullet had gone clean through his neck. Although he was losing blood at an alarming rate, he obstinately refused our offer to dress his wounds. Judging by his expression, he despised the use of bandages to stem the blood. On being offered a rough bed of sacking, he declined it with scorn choosing rather to stand at the back of our open truck, gripping the roof of the driving-hood with both hands, while balancing on his feet as we hit the pot holes. As the Sun rose, he stared at it, as if he were hypnotised. Before long, not only had all bleeding stop-ped, but there were only two small dried scabs left to show where the bullet had entered and left his neck. All this had happened within one hour of sunrise. By now, the young Gurage was smiling triumphantly at our obvious be-wilderment to his indifference to pain or loss of blood; not to mention his ability to heal his own wounds within an hour. After another two and a half hours driving, we offered to take him to the British military hospital in Addis Ababa; but, with a croaking laugh, he refused. We asked ourselves, 'How can a man laugh, who has just been shot through the neck?" Finally, he even expressed a few words of thanks, before coolly sauntering off, as if he had just been on holiday.'

Physical Healing

Matter is energy, and all our activities in this world can be seen as no more than re-arranging the energy patterns according to the dictates of our pralabd karma or destiny. We take pride in or identify with what we do; we may build it up in our minds to be something of importance or value to ourselves or to humanity. But in reality, we are just puppets in the great cosmic energy dance.

Both 'good' and 'bad' activities are necessary for the continuance of life in this physical world. If we had only 'good' or 'bad' karmas, we would not be here, we would be in regions of 'all-good' or 'all-bad' vibration.

The work of the various healing arts can be seen in the same light. Whether it is modern, conventional medicine and surgery or more esoteric forms of healing, with roots in subtle energy balancing, the applied therapy does no more than re-arrange the energy patterns of the body, mind and emotions in order to create harmony and health, ease rather than disease.

The tendency to criticize or be mistrustful of areas of healing that one does not understand needs therefore to be sublimated. Often the unconventional, alternative therapist is as rigid in his stance as the conventional medical mind. There is no reason why the best of both worlds should not work together for the benefit of humanity.

Healing, after all, is the declared intention of all practitioners. One's personal prejudices, fears and jealousies must at least be recognized and resisted. It is too easy and too human to simply criticize that which we do not understand.

In Chinese hospitals, both modern medicine and ancient Chinese natural (herbal) medicine and acupuncture, work side by side. There is a time and place for both. There are people who would prefer one to the other. We cannot make up our minds on the basis of prejudice as to what is best for a patient. There is always room for improvement in our own style of healing, and a doctor must also know how to listen to his patient.

Each person is a unique individual and needs individual, loving care to be brought back to, or maintained, in a condition of health and well-being. The human qualities and depth of understanding of the practitioner are also of paramount importance. Such depth of personality and even spirituality cannot be taught in the lecture hall, but have to be developed within the individual student. The system of medicine has to have a structure in which this love and care can be encouraged. There are many good conventional doctors who simply do not have the time or resources even to get to know their patients, while many alternative therapists will spend an hour or an hour and a half with a new patient, a luxury few medical doctors can afford.

Generally speaking, the division between alternative and conventional medicine lies in the holistic or whole person approach of the alternative practitioner, with the emphasis upon the maintenance of health and well-being, rather than the symptomatic palliation of the negative outward conditions or disease. This world is essentially imperfect and therefore a pragmatic and practical approach to problems more usually results in a harmonious solution, rather than the intense application of philosophical ideologies beyond the bounds of everyday practicality.

Let me create a simple scenario:

A person is involved in a major accident and breaks a leg, perhaps incurring multiple fractures. He is in pain and there are also serious flesh wounds. The ambulance arrives on the scene. The trained personnel administer, perhaps a homoeopathic remedy, or a subtle flower essence, for the shock and emotional trauma. They keep him warm with blankets. They use a homoeopathic or herbal ointment for both the flesh wounds and the pain. An acupuncturist may also help to alleviate the pain. If the pain is too intense, then perhaps the moment is correct for a painkilling drug. The patient is taken to the hospital. The casualty surgeon is called and the antiseptic theatre is prepared. The patient requires anaesthetic, perhaps acupuncture, maybe a modern drug, perhaps a herbal substitute. If a drug is administered, then the doctor knows that he will have to deal with the side effects later. Right now, it is the most practical possibility available.

The surgeon works on the fracture, he may use traction or even stainless steel pins to hold the structure in place. X-rays will be of help in seeing more clearly the nature of the fracture. The flesh wounds are treated – there are many wonderfully curative herbal and homoeopathic preparations that can be used as packs and poultices. Stitches may be required. The leg is set in plaster.

The patient rests. According to the nature of the individual, homoeopathic, herbal, acupuncture, subtle energy essences such as flower remedies are used to strengthen the dis-harmonized body, mind and emotions of the patient and boost his natural resources. His diet is carefully considered. Top quality fuel is required to restore the body-machine to full health.

The emotional and psychological aspects of the accident are discussed in a wholesome manner with trained and caring staff. The patient slowly recovers and is eventually discharged, with considerable further healing of the leg yet to take place. An osteopath may be consulted to check for any spinal mal-adjustments. Physiotherapy may be required to help bring full movement back into the limb. Subtle energy balancing techniques, herbs and dietary considerations will all help to restore our patient to full health and well-being. In our ideal scenario, he probably receives so much loving care that he is never the same again and as a human being, has benefited inestimably from his accident.

And so on. The potential negative has been turned into positive. The point is, of course, that all aspects of the injured person are considered and nourished, not just the leg, and that all therapies and therapists work together without personal prejudice. It all seems so common-sensical and yet there are few hospitals or healing centres where such treatment can be found or even envisaged.

There is a right time and place and circumstance for everything. There is no reason why modern scientific practices should not work hand in hand with ancient or modern holistic and natural methods. A doctor or therapist cannot be expected to know everything about all healing methods. Everybody is a specialist, he reflects his own capabilities and nature in his work. The multitalented are rare. What is required amongst healers is a knowledge of the full spectrum of healing possibilities: *to know when someone else will be of more value to a patient than oneself.*

We are all different and are attuned in different ways. Certain forms of treatment will resonate naturally with certain people and be the correct therapy for them. They will both accept it mentally and feel the benefits. Other treatments will be better for other people. The alignment of thought with practice, a belief in what one is doing – faith – is also of importance. It is quite well-known that the mind can effect physiological functioning as well as vice-versa. Good treatment and faith in that treatment go hand in hand. The mind is very powerful: mental energy is directly connected to emotional and physical energies.

Healing with surgery or drugs is a manipulation of gross physical energy patterns or molecular structures. Often, no-one really knows how a drug has the effect it does. Being mostly of foreign nature, side-effects are bound to occur. The subtle energy aspects are largely ignored. The dissonance created in cellular, molecular, sub-atomic, etheric, emotional and mental energies will be felt as general malaise, as 'not feeling too good'. If drugs or surgery are the only possibility for treatment as in an accident or severe bacterial or viral infection etc. – then the subtle disharmonies created need to be considered at the same time or as soon as practical.

Non-toxic, herbal remedies, being of more natural origin are more in tune with the natural processes of the body. But everything too has a subtle energy aspect which is attuned to the intentions of the administrators. The intentions of the humans involved are all present in the remedy. 'Green fingers' does not apply only to gardeners! If the prime motivation behind the creation of a drug or remedy is profit; if the doctor administers without careful consideration; if there is a lack of long-sightedness and caring love in the process at any stage, it will be reflected in the results. This is true of all aspects of life, not just healing. Love works wonders. Care, consideration, thoughtfulness, harmony – they all leave a nourishing influence in subtle energy patterns. We need 'green fingers' in all human relationships.

Care and love in its preparation and administration will make a remedy work for one therapist while another, without such qualities, may not get the same results. Ideally, treatment has to be correct at all levels: the right treatment, given at the right time, with the right attitude of mind. The patient, too, has his part to play in the process; he cannot remain passive and expect health and well-being to descend on him without personal effort.

Homoeopathic and flower essence remedies consist almost entirely of the subtle energy vibration resonant with the condition they seek to balance – physical, mental and/or emotional. Similarly, with certain crystal energies, either within the crystal itself or transmitted to pure water as a subtle energy vibration – these being the gem remedies now available. The quality of preparation, the subtle energy and intentions of those involved in the manufacture of the remedies will reflect in their efficacy. A meal prepared with love and concentration will produce happiness amongst those who eat it. It will also improve the flavour. A meal prepared with anger and resentment will create divisions amongst those who eat it. The process is the same throughout all human activity. The way things are done is as important as the deeds themselves.

Acupuncture and acupressure (Shiatsu) represent the most intricately mapped of all subtle energy therapies. The flow of subtle energies and their relationship to physiological as well as to emotional and mental energies is represented as a detailed science, the results of which can be profound. When scientists 'discover', for example, that the use of acupuncture to create local anaesthesia, creates endomorphins which, they say, 'cause' the anaesthesia, they are missing the point. The endomorphins are a secondary aspect, part of the effect of subtle energy manipulation, not the primary cause.

The ability simultaneously to hold in mind both the concepts of horizontal and vertical energy spectra must be developed to begin to understand cosmic energy pathways and their interconnections and relationships. Horizontal energies affect each other in a 'sideways' manner. Vertical energies are derived out of each other and are inherently bound together both upwards and downwards.

Radionics therapy works entirely at the subtle energy levels and can hence be used for healing at a distance. All that is required is a tuning device. Some personal part of the patient to provide the resonance and medium for communication – a hair, a blood-spot, a photograph, a signature – anything that contains the unique vibration of the individual. Even some modern physicists are developing theories which require that all energy be instantaneously interconnected at a pre-sub-atomic (or subtle) level, regardless of spatial differentiation. The communication gap between physics and mysticism is rapidly closing.

This multitude of healing arts and their therapists can be thought of like an orchestra of different instruments and their musicians. No musician is expected to have such a gift that he can play all the instruments; he will play the one to which he is the most drawn and naturally gifted. Some may play more than one, only a small few are so talented that many types of instrument are within their capabilities. But all the musicians understand, to one degree or another, the place and importance of the other musicians and instruments. The flute soloist will never suggest that he plays the part of the pianist. No true musician will attempt to exclude a new talent from the orchestra, at least without giving it an unbiased ear. Maybe it is a bent tin whistle, played badly by an amateur and best omitted! Perhaps, it is a simple steel drum, but played with finesse by the West Indian musician. Or maybe it is a new and powerful instrument that causes feelings of jealousy and threatens the position of the first violin, but must be included for the benefit of the total music. It could be that the new instrument is beautiful but strange – like the Indian sitar when first heard by Western ears – and needs its own context to be successful. Some instruments indeed are best in a solo role – the piano and guitar, for instance, backed up, perhaps, by the full weight of the orchestra.

There are many points that can be drawn from this analogy. The orchestra is a microcosm of life as well as the healing arts. And from analogies that carry no emotional or personal charge, we can assess our own views and degree of tolerance, love and understanding for our fellow human beings and their activities. The history of medicine and healing is replete with battles between the humans involved. The battles are normally fought in the *name* of orthodoxy and human safety, though the real nature of the fight is more frequently that of human pride, obstinacy, ego and profit.

Let me give one example taken from Barbara Griggs' compelling history of herbalism, *Green Pharmacy*. Tens of thousands of British Sailors died of scurvy due to lack of vitamin C until in 1795, the British Admiralty finally declared that every sailor should have a ration of one ounce of lemon juice, issued after his sixth week at sea. After that, scurvy became something of the past to the British Navy. However, as early as 1593, John Hawkins wrote of the curative powers of *'Sowre Orange and Lemons'* John Wood- hall's *Surgion's Mate*, published in 1617, was in every ship surgeon's cabin, wherein he says 'the use of the juice of Lemons is a precious medicine and well tried, being sound and good, let it have the chiefe place for it will deserve it.' The Dutch Navy suffered little from scurvy because Sauer- kraut, which contains vitamin C, was a regular part of their diet. 'Unqualified' London street doctors, who needed success to survive, all had extracts of scurvy grass for sale, or the herb itself. Scurvy grass, which contains a reasonable quantity of vitamin C, at that time grew along the banks of the Thames and all around the east coast of England.

Meanwhile, the orthodox medical profession established such theories as: scurvy was a new disease sent by God as a punishment for the sins of the world (Eugalero, 1641); it was caused by unwholesome air, and either a 'sulphureo- saline' or else a 'salino-sulphureous dyscrasy of the blood' (Dr. Willis, 1667); the cause was 'an extraordinary separ- ation of the serous part of the blood from the crassamen- tum' (Boerheave, 17th Century). 'Cures' ranged from repeated bleedings and coolings, warming remedies, purges, deobstruents (open the bowels and pores), to mercury – the latter abruptly terminating the lives of the sufferers.

The British Navy had no provision for fresh vegetables or fruit in the diet of its sailors and only more enlightened captains provided this diet. During the Seven Years War with France and Spain, 130,000 of the 185,000 men pressed into service with the navy died of disease, the majority from scurvy.

Finally, in 1747, the naval surgeon James Lind conducted his own trial, based on extensive research and the results of his *experimental* research on twelve scurvy patients to whom he gave either cider, a preparation of garlic and gum myrrh, elixir of vitriol, vinegar, sea water or two oranges and a lemon per day. After two weeks, those on cider were a little better while the two on oranges and lemons were back on their feet. The rest showed very little, if any, signs of recovery.

Lind presented his case with every possible piece of information he could find, both current and historical, concluding that: 'Experience indeed sufficiently shows, that as greens or fresh vegetables with ripe fruits, are the best remedies for it, so they prove the most effectual preservative against it.'

Even so, *it took another fifty years* and many more deaths before the admiralty finally acknowledged the evidence and ordered the inclusion of lemon juice into sailors' diet.

The 'moral' of the story is very clear. The difficulty is that prejudice never appears as such to us, when we are under its influence. We always present it to ourselves and others in different disguises, with rational justifications – and the personal, self-interested, sub-conscious but powerful motives remain hidden from all but those with an eye of understanding. This is unfortunately the nature of the human mind!

Vibrational Aspects of Disease

A recent ten day trip to Delhi brought home to me once again the power of vibrational disturbance in the manifestation of disease. I am not a person to get ill, in fact until this trip, I had not even had a cold for over a year. And whenever a cold strikes, it is normally all over within a week. However while getting into my car at 6.30a.m. to drive down to Heathrow Airport in London, I felt the first twinges of a sore throat – with myself as with many others, a pre-cursor to the ordinary common cold.

I felt fine and during the flight the throat did not develop, if anything it subsided. It was an easy ten hour trip and we were in our hotel by 8.00p.m., British time, 1.30a.m. Delhi time. Anyone who has been to Delhi knows that the vibration and atmosphere of the place is wildly different from the orderliness of Britain or America. It is dirty, dusty, noisy and packed with people, many of them living in their street hovels of makeshift coverings. Delhi has some pretty smelly areas too – we called one of the places we visited: 'The House at Pooh Corner'!

For foreigners, Delhi has a wide variety of coughs, colds, 'flus and tummy bugs, all with their own unmistakable Indian flavour of throat conditions, head and body feelings. If you have been to India, you will know what I am talking about. An Indian cold is different from a British one in the way it gets you!

I however, had brought a 'British' cold with me. My wife Farida and I were not jet-lagged and our circadian rhythms adjusted rapidly to the five and a half hour time difference. The new vibration of our environment, however, made us feel somewhat out of kilter, the sense of dislocation not an altogether unpleasant feeling, but rather akin to a easy detachment from our surroundings.

It was clear however, that the change in vibration was now encouraging the cold, which came on with an Indian, not British, flavour after an unusually drawn out sore-throat phase of about five days. It was not a lasting affair, the peak only spanning a day and a half. Our visit was a short one and by the last day of our trip, it was practically over.

The flight home was not so easy. We left for the airport in the middle of the night at 1.30a.m. after only three hours sleep. The flight was somehow more disharmonious, physically. Sleep was a stranger to me and the aeroplane felt electrostatically and magnetically more disorienting. We arrived back at Heathrow, mid-morning British time, and motored home to Cambridge.

My cold now began to develop once again, this time with characteristically British touches. You have to believe me on this, the symptoms are, of course, subjective. This time, the effects of the flight were more apparent – travellling west to east – and the change in the environmental vibration back to British, though welcome, was once again un-settling. This time the cold took nearly ten days of mucus and mildly feverish symptoms to disappear.

Now the reason I am going into all this is because it

became very clear to me that the cold I was experiencing was a manifestion of the body's adjustment to changing vibrations in the subtle atmosphere of the environment. Its ups and downs were directly related to where I was – India or England. And it brought to mind the fact that colds and 'flus, at least in myself, are most commonly experienced in Spring, Autumn or when on holiday in another country, especially after an aeroplane flight. The vibrational change in the atmosphere due to the change in seasons is really quite marked. You may well have noticed yourself how Spring suddenly feels to have arrived, even though the process of change is gradual. Over a relatively short period, the mood of nature has moved into the rhythm of new life. Similarly with Autumn, the leaves may have shown signs of turning for some while, but almost abruptly one morning, you suddenly feel the in-drawing nostalgia of Autumn filter into your awareness and you know that summer is over – even if the weather is warm, sometimes, in England, warmer than summer itself.

Nature moves in these rhythms and these atmospheres are responded to and augmented by all the living creatures. In Spring, they mate and build their nests while energy is outwardly vibrant and joyous. In Autumn, energy is conserved and drawn in. Plants and trees withdraw to their roots, some animals hibernate. Energy is concentrated within. Autumn is a time of sweet nostalgia, of contented melancholy. In more tropical climates, like India, the physical change of seasons can be very pronounced, almost to the day. And with the change in seasons come the coughs and colds – the body's response to its relationship to a change in vibration. Other diseases may not be directly attributable to a change in season or vibration, but the 'cold' definitely is.

Busy people, too, often get their colds at weekends! It seems unfair, but then the connection of mind, emotions and body are not so obscure to us as to provide no understanding of this phenomenon. I have many friends who say quite simply that they have no time to 'catch a cold'!

Of course, I am aware of the conventional, viral explanation of a cold and I do not dispute the biochemical and pathological facts. But it is, I believe a part of the outworking of energy patterns. The subtle energy vibrations at the root of a cold obviously have to manifest themeslves in energy disturbances at the molecular and biochemical level. And, no doubt, a cold can be 'caught' – but only when there is a vibrational element within the 'catcher', that allows the virus (or bacteria) to take root.

Immunology may be interested to look at things from this point of view and, indeed, homoeopathic nosodes and antidotes to specific illnesses have been worked out along these lines. Create healing strength and immunity at the subtle level and the biochemical system of antibodies and so on, automatically falls into place, creating natural resistance to disease.

This change of vibrational atmosphere also provides us with an understanding of 'new' diseases, such as AIDS. The disease has its roots in our environmental and socio-logical subtle energy conditions, allowing the existence of the virus as an effect not a prime cause, in the vertical energy spectrum of its existence. This explains why not everbody shows symptoms of the virus, even if it is absorbed into their blood stream. In fact, no disease can be contracted if there is no element in the subtle make-up of the individual with which it can resonate.

While on our Indian trip, Farida remained free of the cold I mentioned until, one day, feeling depressed, she allowed the negative aspects of India's vibrations to get into her mind. The next day, she awoke with a sore throat and the knowledge that she had herself opened the doors to the cold.

After reading this section, she added: 'Bach flower remedies and homoeopathic medication defer treatment of disease or symptoms to the higher plane of personality groups of vibrational similarity. The state of mind precedes the illness, disturbs the physical body and is the true cause of the disease. The different personality types respond to illness in a similar way, even though they have different symptoms. One becomes vulnerable when vibrational changes of travel, new cultures and climate affect one's being. Each individulal responds according to personality type – for example with fear, uncertainty, guilt, pride etc. As soon as one's mind goes out of balance the doorway to the onset of uncomfortable symptoms is open. The recognition and conscious awareness of the first disturbances in mental and emotional life become more and more clear until an individual can prevent illness by treating the mind. Dr Bach also taught that one could correct early stages of illness merely by thinking of the remedy and restoring balance.'

I can well recall when Farida first came to England. She is Canadian, but had moved to California and Arizona in her early twenties, where for the first time in her life she began to feel well, and vibrant with health. The hot, dry desert atmosphere, beloved by many, has a special healing vibration and she blossomed. Nearly twenty years later, when I 'imported' her to damp, cold England, she received such a shock of vibration, as well as of culture, that it took many years for her to acclimatize. In fact, I would say that it took almost seven years. Every cell and molecule in her body was vibrating with the Arizona and Californian desert atmosphere. Physiologically she was totally thrown out of step and emotionally too, and this vibrant being now struggled to keep her head afloat.

In fact, it was only when Dr. Yao came to stay with us, seven and a half years after her arrival in England, giving us a series of very powerful Pulsor®, energy balancing treatments (see chapter 5) that she finally felt attuned to England. The pull of cellular attachment to the desert finally left and her body felt at home here, at last.

Another friend of ours, born and bred in India in a British family, had to leave at the time of partition in 1945 and come to England, an alien land. The clarity and spirituality in the atmosphere of the Indian Himalayan hill stations, where her family home was situated – as well as amid the towns and villages – is powerful, reflecting the centuries of mystic and yogic philosophy and thinking inherent among India's peoples. This atmosphere is not totally obscured today, even amidst the squalid areas of poverty-stricken urban environments.

This friend, like Farida, was hit by the change in atmosphere between the two countries and even now, after a lapse of forty years, her affinity with India is as strong as ever, though the body and mind have long since adapted as much as they may.

This quality of subtle vibration, then, is an inherent environmental factor in our states of well-being and disease, never to be neglected in any serious healing work. It is more difficult to quantify – indeed the totally analytical scientific approach will have a hard time getting to grips with this ever changing and fluid energy dance. But then, can one really expect to capture life under a microscope?

CHAPTER 4

Energy, Polarity and Harmony

Modern man is by now well acquainted with the fact that the physical universe as perceived by our five senses is very different in appearance to that which is described by science. This scientific description has changed and is continually changing.

Other species inhabiting this planet have senses which we do not have, in their perception of physical matter: some birds have a sense which perceives the magnetic grid of the earth and they use it for migration. Other creatures perceive wavelengths and frequencies of sound and electromagnetic energy (eg. light) that we cannot. Dogs, horses, elephants and probably most other animals seem to have a 'sixth sense' – they are aware of the subtle energy vibrations of both humans and their fellow creatures. If you have children – or you may remember it from your own school days – the span of time between archaeologists' estimates of the age of the earliest known fossils and the first fossil evidence of man is often to be seen festooned around the classroom on the scale of a large toilet roll, with Man's existence normally acknowledged to be little more than the width of the final serrated edge! Whether you care to believe such flimsy evidence in its entirety is up to the individual, but it does give one an idea of relative scales.

Similarly, if the whole of the electromagnetic spectrum were compared to a distance of a thousand miles (a little more than the distance from Land's End to John O'Groats by road, the length of England and Scotland), then the range of visible wavelengths which we call light, and perceive through our physical eyes, would measure as a distance of about a half of one billionth of an inch, (one billion equalling one thousand million).

Furthermore, even amongst humans, we differ in both our perceptive abilities and in our interpretation of the perceived data! Some people have a far higher frequency range in their hearing than others, some are colour-blind, an artist sees colours more vividly, musicians may have 'perfect pitch', some have altogether lost one or more of their senses, while an increasing number are tuned to the subtle vibrations of objects and people. Our mood and state of health and well-being also affect our perceptions. In other words, what we perceive is not a fixed reality, but a subjective experience based upon our own physical, emotional and mental make-up.

The proposition then, that there are energy fields and patterns of which we are – through our five regular senses – unaware, should at least be acceptable to us as a working hypothesis. We still switch on our TV and are happy to use a remote control without ever perceiving anything 'coming into' our home or pass from our remote-control device to the TV set! Indeed, we can still use electricity without understanding its nature and governing laws.

Our physical universe is a mixture of both perceivable and imperceivable 'gross' matter and more subtle energy fields. Subtle energy fields are the blueprint of physical matter. Our physical body is actually two bodies. The gross physical body, perceivable by the five normal senses, and the subtle – sometimes called etheric – body of which the physical is a precipitation or reflection downwards. The state of the subtle body determines the health of the physical body. In high energy physics terminology, the subtle energy is the 'ghost' – energy from which physical matter is derived. Some physicists these days talk of 'ghost' electrons, for example. No scientist has ever demonstrated the existence of a 'ghost' electron, but theoretically, its existence would seem to be essential to scientific thinking and rationality. In Nature, you cannot get 'something' for 'nothing', for an electron or any sub-atomic particle to exist, there must be something to substantiate it, or give it its energy. That is its 'ghost' or subtle counterpart.

As we described in the mystic cosmology, the universe is said to be the play of the Creator. Mystics say that the Source is One. That means: no movement, no differentiation, just perfect peace and oneness, bliss and love. Creation is an act, or movement within the One. He is still one and at peace, say the mystics. But within Himself, He has created a game of love with Himself, His creation is like the froth on his periphery. These are indeed only metaphors to describe a reality which is best experienced.

However one cares to describe it, motion and differentiation in the energy fields of the cosmos are its basis for existence. And this game of movement is held together through the action of the three states or attributes of mind and matter, the gunas, as described in the prologue. Some of their aspects may be listed as follows:

Rajas (Yang)	*Satvas*	*Tamas (Yin)*
Action	Rest	Inaction
Positive	Zero/Neutral	Negative
Expansion	Equilibrium	Compression
Above	Mid-point	Below
Forward	Motionless	Backwards
Centrifugal	In Orbit	Centripetal
Birth	Living	Death
Day	Dawn/Dusk	Night
Anabolism	Metabolism	Catabolism

As discussed previously, all the attributes of life and creation can be seen in these terms. Indeed, the interplay of these forces is an underlying reality in all existence. Actually, it is impossible to define one activity as entirely related to the activity of one guna. Everything contains within it the seeds (at least) of other gunas, for it is impossible to have a one-sided coin, a 'yes' without an implied 'no', an up without a down. So when we say that something is rajas, it means that the rajas aspect is in the ascendant, at that time. And since all energy interchanges have innumerable aspects – indeed the aspects themselves have aspects (this is getting like little fleas and bigger fleas!) – some aspects may be rajas and some tamas, while others may be in balance, or satvas. And since, in fact, 'there is just one big thing going on', we can say that within *that*, the principle of duality or the gunas or yin and yang hold sway.

Note, especially, that the guna of rest is actually a state of balance or tension between opposing forces, an equilibrium between the positive and the negative. Therefore, it is not a state of real peace. The balance can be upset at any time. Within the spheres of movement and creation it is desirable, but true peace is beyond the gunas, beyond the realms of mind and matter, firmly rooted in the Source.

Furthermore, balance and rest are relative, as our old friend Einstein was quick to point out. We may be at rest on our planet, but relative to the sun, our earth is rocketing through space at many miles per second. Thus, what is positive for one may be negative for another. And this is due entirely to the complexity of the energy currents and fields in which we are deeply entangled, both within and without.

In the Bhagavad Gita, the gunas are also spoken of as the 'pairs of opposites'. Bear them with equanimity, Krishna advises his disciple Arjuna. Equanimity means finding the balance-point, the middle guna between them, steering a true and noble path through life.

Now, within the energy fields of our physical universe, and observed from a sub-atomic, as well as subtle point of view, these three forces can be constantly seen in action. We have the cohering forces of gravity, magnetism and energy moving in a clockwise spiral – the innate attraction of energy for energy, matter for matter. And we have the tendency to expand and move apart, the centrifugal force of energy moving in an anti-clockwise motion.

All sub-atomic particles are in constant motion, they spin and move in three dimensions. One can say that the movement of energy in three dimensions is what makes physical matter 'solid' or 'real'. This physical universe is motion, action, cause and effect – *karma* as the Indian yogis and mystic philosophers call it.

The nature of this movement, including the attraction and repulsion of forces within atomic structure is one of the key areas of research in modern physics. It becomes clear, therefore that the link-point between subtle energy fields and their first manifestation, crystallization or precipitation as gross physical matter will be in the nature of the movement and spin of sub-atomic energy. Gross matter is simply more subtle matter stepped down in its vibratory rate in the heirarchy of creative energy – froth on the froth, so to speak. And within this movement, are discovered the outworking of the gunas – the three basic forces of nature.

All forces and movement therefore have polarity, there cannot be an up without a down, a plus without a minus, a 'yes' without a 'no'. This is true both conceptually, in our thinking, as well as in the processes of nature. And since our gross physical bodies consist of sub-atomic matter, of energy in motion, patterned and shaped into the molecular, physiological and anatomical structures and processes that we know of as a living body, it more or less goes without saying that these positive and negative aspects will be reflected in sub-atomic motion and being.

This basic *polarity* in our body-emotion-mind complex has been used by innumerable therapies throughout the ages, both consciously and unconsciously, for the maintenance of good health and the combating of disease. Our gross physical body is the manifestation of its more subtle 'counterpart' and the polarities and state of balance in the one will directly effect the state of balance within the other. When energy flows, it moves from plus to minus, from high to low, to create equilibrium. But for existence to continue the polarity must be maintained in order for the energy flow to continue. In electricity, we use a battery or a generator, in magnetism a north and a south pole and at a deeper level in sub-atomic matter, we have movement and the forces of attraction and repulsion. All of these *polarities* are necessarily reflections of polarities at more subtle levels.

Note too, that polarities can and do change without loss of energy. When you bounce a ball against a wall, its direction changes, but not so the energy content of the event. Thus, an environmental change which causes a change in the harmony and spin of sub-atomic matter will automatically change the polarities within the subtle energy fields and vice versa, without any external visible signs of this change in state. In other words, the inner state of kinetic being within sub-atomic matter can vary without the five normal human senses being able to perceive any difference.

In our bodies, the state of our subtle energy determines our degree of physical health and emotional/mental well-being. In our environment, the harmony or disharmony within subtle energy and the sub-atomic energy patterns, gives rise to the experience of good or bad atmospheres or vibrations. Our physical bodies, then, are comprised of the gross physical of which we are easily aware and the subtle or etheric, the blueprint of the physical, which controls our state of health in the gross physical. Healing can therefore take place in two directions – by controlling the gross physical which will change the polarities in the subtle and/or by changing the polarities in the subtle which will reflect downwards and manifest as the creation of healthy tissues in the gross physical. In practice, those involved in the healing professions, consciously or unconsciously use a mixture of both.

An acupuncturist, for example, will work on the subtle fields, but may also recommend the use of certain herbs, as well as changes in diet, lifestyle and mental attitude to compliment his work in the subtle energy fields. He may also give a spinal manipulation for back sufferers if he is so trained, whilst also being able to manipulate the structure of the spine purely through his work with needles on the subtle body. Depending upon the circumstances, one approach may be more appropriate than another.

Furthermore, just as there are myriad forms in the physical world and physiological systems within our body, so too are there a multitude of vibratory rates or patterns within subtle energy. Some can be considered as 'horizontal', or at the same energy level; others are 'vertical' or 'inward', in the sense that they are the blueprint and lower energies are derived from them – in just the same way that the physical objects which make up our everyday world of gross matter are energy fields and particles, when looked at from the sub-atomic point of view.

Therefore, there are many subtle energy healing systems, each working on different, but allied, energy fields. Some are worked out in great detail, such as acupuncture; others adopt a simpler approach and often rely to a great degree upon the finer perceptions, intuition and innate healing gift of the practitioner.

Sub-Atomic Spin and Magnetism

The idea that spin direction is related to the essential duality, the interplay of positive and negative forces is not unique. We find it, for example, in the writings of Davis and Rawls, two pioneers of research into the effect of magnetism on the human body. They discovered that the magnetic poles, North and South, have differing properties and effects on living organisms. To quote from their book, *The Magnetic Effect*: 'We were able to report this discovery by the actual measurement of the direction of the electron spin that is transmitted from the two poles of all magnets.

'Further, the direction of the movement of the electrons (magnetic energy) in the North and South poles was reverse in nature. In fact, energy coming from the South pole of a magnet moved, travelled and took on a spinning vortex of energy to the right or clockwise, while that energy coming from the North pole of a magnet spun, moved and cycled to the left or counterclockwise.

'This discovery was not confirmed officially until the development of the present space age and the actual magnetic measurements that were made by complex technical magnetometers from space. The energy of a magnet, like that of the earth's two magnetic poles, the North and South poles, does not simply leave one pole and travel around the magnet to re-enter the other end of the magnet, but on leaving the South pole, it travels only half way around the magnet to its centre. Here it alters its electronic spin, taking on a reverse spin and resultant form of energy, and leaves the centre of the magnet or earth to continue on, re-entering the North pole of the magnet or earth, as the case may be. Published space research reports now prove this to be fact.' Indeed, scientists have long been aware that single electrons themselves behave like magnets.

Davis and Rawls actually developed a method of photographing 'these invisible lines of force.' They 'were able to see the two spinning vortexes of magnetic energy and examine them in detail.' This work is described in their book: *Magnetism and Its Effect of the Living System.*

Ball Lightning and Particle Spin

A breakthrough (in 1985) by Dr Geert Dijkhuis, director of a Rotterdam based company, offers some hope of using particle spin as part of a new energy source. Dr Dijkhuis' research has centred on the artificial creation of ball lightning, both as a means of understanding its nature and utilizing its energies. Ball lightning has traditionally been discarded by scientists as folk lore, until continuing reports of these luminous electric spheres that can float around inside vehicles, houses and even aeroplanes after lightning storms, has brought their existence into the laboratory for understanding. In fact, some while ago, ball lightning was observed by the amazed and fascinated eyes of a physicist travelling in a aeroplane, who later wrote up his experience, published in a scientific journal – I forget which one unfortunately, I believe it was the *New Scientist*.

Dr Dijkhuis has succeeded in producing a 10cm variant of ball lightning, lasting just one second, hoping to produce a larger three second ball, within the year. Dr Dijkhuis, whose doctorate in applied physics is from Stanford University, theorizes that ball lightning consists of super-conducting ionized gas, ionized by proximity to a lightning bolt, and forming itself into vortices, which spin in the same direction as the particles of which they consist. This spin is then transmitted to the whole, creating a spinning luminous ball.

Dr Dijkhuis' vision is that this work could lead to a relatively small nuclear reactor running on deuterium, obtainable from sea water and of course, considerably cheaper and safer than conventional nuclear fuels.

Subtle Energy Terminology

Throughout the literature on subtle energy topics, we encounter a wide variety of names used in its description. Just as the physical universe displays an endless show of shifting and changing energy patterns, part of which we discern through our senses, so too in the subtle energy fields do we find a spectrum of energies. Different therapies seem to deal with different aspects or areas of these energies. Being beyond our five physical senses, they are more difficult to chart and the names used to describe them can become confusing. We use 'subtle energy' to describe all subtle physical and super-physical energies up to the level of mental or thought vibrations. Other terms, some specific, some general are: etheric, Ch'i, prana, bio-energy, auric force field, vortex energy and many more.

It also needs to be pointed out quite clearly that there is a potential semantic difficulty in the use of the terms *positive* and *negative*. These terms, actually, have two meanings. Sometimes they are used as a value judgement – negative emotions and thoughts, for example, or a negative personality and attitude. Sometimes they are used in reference to an aspect of polarity where no value judgement is implied – negative electrical charge, for example. These are the words used in our language to express these ideas and the meaning should normally be clear from the context. Sometimes there is a mixture of meaning, but as long as one is aware of the different uses of the word, there should be no confusion.

The Mind – Emotion – Body Complex

Nature's polarities are expressed in many ways within living creatures. From the highest point of view, the soul is the creative, positive current, while the Universal Mind is the neutral and the physical universe the negative pole of creation. Within our human constitution, the energy of our physical thought or thinking mind represents the positive pole, the emotions – our intermediate energies – largely finding expression as unconscious energy – are the neutral pole, while the gross physical matter of our body is the negative pole.

These energies are reflected in the physical organs over which they preside and find expression. Thus the mind reflects in the brain, the sense organs and in the throat through speech. These are the centres of intelligence and control within the body, the throat centre or chakra being the seat of the most subtle of the five tattwas or elements, that or 'ether' or akash, out of which the other elements are formed, while the sixth chakra or Do-dal-Kanwal, situated behind the eyes, is the centre at which concentration of the mental faculties is first attempted in the meditative process of ascent to higher or inner regions. The mental energies and their outward manifestation are thus the controllers, the positive pole from which energy flows for the creation and control of lower energies and structures.

The self-possessed person is the one who is gathered together behind his eyes. He has the most control of himself and can be a leader of others if he is so constituted. To be self-possessed requires honesty, love and a high moral character, in harmony with Natural Law. The dishonest man is shifty-eyed, we say. His focus of being is scattered. He can never meet the eyes of an honest man. His ego and self-desire force his attention to lower, more unconsious levels within his body and he is hardly aware of himself as a living, conscious entity. Honesty is an attribute of the akash element, situated in the throat centre and pure honesty is something very few of us possess, our egos always leading us astray to one degree or another.

In yogic practice, as the yogi concentrates on the centres within the body and develops his consciousness at these centres, he attains a mastery of the element associated with that centre. This inner understanding gives him the power to perform miracles – to move solid objects at the rectal chakra that controls the manifestation of the earth element, to walk on water at the next higher, sacral, watery centre, and so on. At the throat centre, the last of the 'Riddhis and Siddhis', the miraculous powers, comes to the yogi. Now his mind is so pure that he is true and honest and everything he says comes out to be true. We say: 'Truth has a ring to it.' It has a power, it reaches our hearts and minds when we hear it. Insincerity is immediately detectable by the honest man. In one whose consciousness is elevated by spiritual practice, truth, love, ego-forgetfulness and true self-possession are manifest in strength of being. Confidence, indeed, is a quality not of brashness, but of a forgetfulness of self, with the mind and soul centred on the Divine.

These then are some aspects of mental energies in our human constitution.

Our emotions are mind energy moving outwards and reflecting against or interacting with the chakras and subtle tattvic fields. This involves the lungs, the circulatory control organ of the heart and the energy centre of the involuntary, unconscious nervous system – the solar plexus as well as the liver and spleen. If we are upset emotionally, we can attain some measure of control by breathing deeply. 'Take a deep breath,' we say. One major problem with emotionally upset people is heart disease. Patients are often given medication to keep them calm, because emotional upset can bring on a heart attack. Fear, an associate of the fire element, has its roots in the solar plexus. We get a knot in the stomach or butterflies. If we eat while we are emotionally upset, our food does not digest, because the fire energy required for digestion and assimilation is being dissipated through our emotional disturbance. It is well known, too, that a fit of anger upsets the functioning of the liver and spleen, also under the control of the fiery element, while emotional upset can bring on a heart attack or cause palpitations

When we get hungry, our attention slips to our stomach, into our emotional centre and away from our rational centre. It is not surprising therefore, that we may get irritable or emotional when needing our meal. Similarly, when tired, the attention slips down to lower centres, the throat centre and lower down and, therefore, once again we are operating in the emotional area of our being and manifest it as anger or other forms of emotional behaviour.

The mind, therefore, directly affects the body through the emotions. The nature of the tattvic activity gives us characteristics that reflect the qualities of those tattwas, as we find in the constitutional types of Ayurvedic medicine, as well as the pattern-finding science of astrology, where personality is directly related to the elemental or tattvic activity.

The lower area of the body is associated with the lower two chakras, through which the material states of water and earth are manifest. These are represented by the sex and water balance organs of the gonads and kidneys and the earthy eliminative function of the rectum.

Sex and emotion are powerfully linked. When, in a relationship, our attention drops to the sex centre, we are in increasing danger of losing our rationality and our attention is dragged forcibly away from its princely centre in our forehead. Indeed, the laws of many countries, tacitly admit this fact when they lay a greater penalty on pre-meditated crimes requiring 'rational' thought than on 'crime passionelle.'

As human beings, we need all the aspects of our constitution to be functioning in harmony. Our body and its gross requirements should be cared for, but not indulged. Our emotional life and feelings need to be in healthy balance – we need a heart to balance our head. And our mental rationality should be tempered with a knowledge of the limitations and real function of the intellect.

There are as many subtle variations in the way these energies manifest themselves as there are humans, for broadly speaking, these are the energies that constitute our physical being. The capable man who makes plans in his

mind and puts them into action has a close coupling
between his mental and physical energies. His emotions
are also closely interwoven between the two and he will
often become impatient and irritable, exhibiting various
aspects of emotional behaviour if he is frustrated in his
attempts to translate his thoughts into action, because he is
also emotionally involved in the successful outcome. The
less that emotional energy is bound up in this complex, the
more rational will be his ability to handle the details and
problems that occur in manifesting his thoughts in physical reality.

The archetype of the hyper-reactive business executive
is one whose mental, emotional and physical energies are
too tightly coupled, often to the detriment of his conscious
rationality. He reacts instinctively and immediately, suffering from high blood pressure, heart attack and stom-
ach-ulcers – outward manifestations of his inner condition.

Using some of the polarity balancing techniques described in the next chapter, one is able to space apart, relax
or loosen the coupling between these energies, thus providing an energy forum in which physical problems will
automatically be relieved and healed.

This example of a business executive is both simple and
also oversimplified. The powerful unconscious emotional
and mental vibrations that make us the way we are and
with which we are born take on innumerable patterns and
are manifested as disease, disharmonious energy patterns
or illness in our physical bodies as a direct reflection of our
personality. We are one energy system. Our physical body
and outer life can be seen as a lower harmonic of our more
inward energies, with all the unconscious complexities of
our personality, finding exact and detailed manifestation in
our state of physical health.

Consider the reverse of the executive – the impractical
idealist who has so many beautiful ideals in mind but has
so loose a coupling to his or her physical energies that little
is ever outwardly accomplished. The painter or musician
working through the higher sense organs of vision and
hearing, in the head, needs another party to find ways of
making a living out of their work. Their hands are finely
sculpted – they may not be the strong square hands of the
intensely practical man. The idealist, the dreamer, is often

emotionally frustrated too because he cannot make things happen according to his mental vision, clouded too with his emotion. But the more placid idealist is a prime target for low blood pressure and poor circulation – his mental, emotional and physical energies being so loosely coupled.

The correlation of specific disease patterns to personality types has been a subject of research in recent years, finding relationships, too, as one would expect, to the personality types described by serious astrology. But Dr Bach many years ago discovered a simple system of medicine, treating always the personality traits with subtle flower essences or energies as a means of correcting imbalances at the higher level.

Body Polarities

Healthy human functioning is achieved when all the natural energy flows that go into the constitution of our being are operating smoothly. Energy flow is the result of polarity, of difference, of a tendency to seek oneness or unity. In this respect, it can be seen that the entire Universe is seeking its Source through a desire to merge and eradicate difference or duality. But the Great Power keeps the play going on and the energy patterns of his creation continue. He is playing the game of seeking Himself, a game of Love. And He alone knows why!

In our mind–emotion–body complex therefore, correct polarity is the essence of well-being and adjustment of polarity is a powerful method of subtle treatment. Harmonize, balance and correct the natural polarities and the concomittant energy flows, and healthy mental, emotional and physical functioning will automatically ensue. How then, is this achieved? The answer is twofold, each connected with the other.

1. By correct living habits.
2. Through external agents – therapy etc.

Correct Living Habits

There are many ways in which this topic can be expressed – moral, philosophical, religious etc. – but since we are maintaining a theme of energy, let us take this as our mode of expression. Working down through the chakras, those all important centres of energy, we start with the eye and throat centres. Here we are concerned with our *mental attitude* and its relationship to our *emotions*, some aspects of which, we have already discussed.

Our attitudes, our approach to life, mentally and emotionally, strongly affect our physical well-being. The energy of our thoughts is at a higher vibratory level than that of our emotions. We say: 'Get a grip on yourself' – we attempt to control our emotions through our rationality. These energies are interconnected – our thoughts or mental vibrations, our emotional energy, our subtle energy and the gross physical. There are energy pathways, linking them. We *think*: 'I will hold up my hand' and via a transformation of energy through to physical levels, we can do so. This is a clear connection and happens automatically and instinctively much of the time. What is also true, but not so readily accepted, is that our thoughts and emotional life are reflected in the state of health or disease of the body. Our subtle energy systems are disharmonized or reversed in polarity by our negative thoughts and emotions, largely sub-conscious, and the manifest result is ill-health and dis-ease. Similarly, a strong, positive attitude and balanced emotional life, lead to good health, well-being and even prosperity.

The level of awareness of an individual depends upon where his inner attention is focused. A person whose attention is totally focused upon his physical body, will identify with it. He will feel that all he is, is his body; that death of the physical body will be the end of him. He is largely unaware of the emotional and mental energy patterns and habits that drive him. He thinks he is free, and yet his true being is so hemmed in by these unconscious, inner habits that he has no more freedom than any other creature of instinct.

A person whose attention rises up to a degree of awareness of their own thoughts and emotions starts asking questions concerning the meaning of their own inner life. As their attention rises, they have spontaneous realizations – 'koans', as Zen Buddhists call them. Meditation increases this awareness, it raises the level of consciousness, it gives a direct insight into the inner workings of one's own mind and being.

Psychological therapy and counselling help to re-arrange these energy patterns of thought and emotion that make up our personality. Poor therapy or certain schools of mind control overdo it. These energies are highly subtle and permit control or dis-orientation of an individual, as in brainwashing techniques.

However, good psychological counselling techniques can lead to an increase in physical health, through the inherent energy pathways via the subtle energy blueprint of physical matter. Meditation is an even better way, since the mental energies automatically find a state of harmony, without the turbidity and confusion of psychotherapy. Each person has to find his own, perhaps pre-destined, path towards self-realization and ultimately God-reali-zation.

Perhaps we should add here that self-realization means the knowledge of the soul when it steps out of the realm of Universal Mind that 'I am THAT', when it knows itself as soul, while still higher up close to the Source itself, the soul exclaims (metaphorically) '*I* do not exist – I am *God*'. Self-realization does not mean just a good knowledge of one's own personality, though this is undoubtedly one of the first steps on the long journey.

Our concern here, however, is to point out the effect on the subtle energies of our inner being. Moreover, since the energy flows both up and down, changes in our subtle energies and harmony at a physical level will reflect up-wards in our mood and thoughts. This indeed, is how food can affect our mind and thoughts, including anaes-thetic drugs, alcohol and psychedelic chemicals. The whole process is highly dynamic and interconnected. It is the vast energy complex we call our life.

Next, we come to the heart and solar plexus centres with their physical manifestions in the organs they super-vise. Here we have the elements of *air* and *fire*. Their balance, too, is essential for the maintenance of correct body polarity.

Air is a conveyor of prana, of vital life energy to our bloodstream and general being. Think of the sparkle and fresh vitality of air laden with prana in the mountains and certain other places, that is so uplifting and invigorating. We intuitively stop and take in deep breaths of it, returning to our urban lives in more vibrant health. Oxygen too, is the fuel for oxidation, out of which comes warmth or fire energy. Air also contains an ionic charge – positive or negative – and all experimentation that has been performed has shown quite conclusively that negative air ionization has marked positive effects on physical health, as well as emotional and mental well-being. This is related back to our discussion of electron spin, its inherent polarity and its role in energy flow within living systems. In electricity, negative charge in the body is associated with strengthening, toning, soothing, refreshing and relaxing, while positive energy is the stimulator and in excess causes pain, irritation, heat and swelling. Together they maintain a polarized balance. It is interesting to note in this respect that researchers into the effects of air ionization on living creatures have noticed that while it is a negative charge that produces long-term enhanced growth in plants, a positive charge will initially cause a sprint in the growth rate, later waning as the plant begins to suffer from energy depletion and 'running on its nerves.'

The two lower chakras oversee the functioning of the watery and earth elements, the assimilation and elimination of our food and drink, the gross body fuel, as well as the procreative functions and sexual energy. The quality and nature of the food and drink that we intake is important to us. Fresh, uncooked live vegetables and fruits, especially sprouts, carry a high level of positive, vital life energy, vibrating within all the cells and molecules. As in all matters, finding the correct balance for oneself is essential. Too much food can create negative conditions in the body as the stomach struggles in overload. Food quality, too, is of importance. Wilted vegetables and poor produce will cause indigestion; similarly with cooked food that is past its prime. Just observing food, one can see when it reaches its tamas guna phase. It seems to radiate a dull aura and vibration.

Water has a particular affinity for subtle energy, both positive and negative and can exert a strong influence on us for good or ill. Look, for example, at the harmonizing effect of a lake or a stream on the surrounding area, while water flowing under a dwelling can cause energy depletion and a negative vibration in the property as the positive energy is withdrawn into the flowing stream.

Pollution

As with many topics constantly in the public eye, this subject has acquired such an emotional content that it is sometimes difficult to consider its rationalities. Pollution is, in essence, a disturbance to the natural flow of energy patterns that is detrimental to the continuance of healthy, vibrant, balanced life. It is, in effect, a negative influence or polarity and almost all pollution that cannot be taken care of by natural processes is created by Man. Animals may not have our propensity for higher consciousness and awareness, but neither are they led astray by negative and selfish intelligence to the extent that they wilfully upset the natural balance for their own personal, short-lived desires and gain. Even the overgrazing of pasture and scrub by such animals as goats, leading to the formation of deserts, is orchestrated by human beings and does not occur in a naturally balanced environment.

Pollution occurs at all levels of human energy and can create negative effects that reflect in energy disturbances within our beings causing ill health and poor quality of life. Advertising and the media are responsible for conscious mental pollution and we are affected too, by the vibrations of other people. Our air and water are polluted by increasing numbers of life-destroying chemicals and inbalances, while our food is often so heavily sprayed, treated, preserved and generally unloved that one is easily able to understand the unhealthy state of the vast majority of humankind. Junk food should indeed carry a government health warning!

Electromagnetic Pollution

This is not a book on environmental care, but one of the areas of pollution that is the most difficult for the conventional scientific community to understand, because of its subtlety, is that of electromagnetic radiation and because of its relevance to our theme and its need for greater exposure, I want to discuss it here.

The body has certain electrical potentials and polarities which will be discussed in the next chapter, and these electrical polarities, probably through the direction of electron spin and certainly through the general harmony, balance and flow of sub-atomic energy movement, affect the polarities and energy flow in our more subtle energy fields. Remember – movement is inherently bound up with polarity. Sub-atomic matter is currently seen by modern physics as energy patterns and forces, vibrating at speeds often approaching that of light. Indeed, this kinetic energy is an inherent aspect of its being. The forces that hold it all together are also an essential part of its existence. These forces are electromagnetic, gravitational and allied fields. Powerful cosmic rays and particle emissions are already known to alter atomic structure even in a macroscopic sense – molecules and atoms are changed permanently – this is part of the effects of radioactive emissions.

It is highly likely, therefore, that all electromagnetic energy, including light, affects the movement of the energy patterns at sub-atomic levels. Since the sub-atomic energy and electromagnetic energy are of the same nature, they will attract and repel; they will interact; they will not be indifferent to each other.

Sub-atomic and electromagnetic energy are amongst the first physical manifestations of subtle energy. The vibrational states of subtle energy will affect the sub-atomic energy patterns and vice versa. Hence it comes as no surprise to find that electromagnetic energy affects the polarities in our subtle body and causes changes in our level of health and well-being. This need not all be negative, however it does seem that it is only the wavelengths of natural sunlight to which our own bodies and systems are attuned. Outside these wavelengths, we start having problems.

Modern man is bombarded by electromagnetic radiation of his own creation. With electrical and magnetic energy reaching us from power lines and cabling, microwave radar and communications, TV and radio broadcasting, industrial and domestic electromagnetic devices, one estimate is of 200 millions times more than our ancestors took in from the sun and cosmic sources. Our body and biophysical energies are receivers, conductors and transmitters of this electromagnetic pollution. If you have ever set up a radio aerial you will know how your own body can also behave as an extension to the aerial, simply by your holding the exposed end of the aerial wire.

You can experiment with one of the modern voltage tracers used by electricians which bleep when within the oscillating electrical induction field created by an alternating current. Place the probe near the mains cable of any electrical appliance and the bleeping rises to a crescendo. If you now hold it near a human hand, the bleeping is normal. But ask the person to hold the cable with their other hand and the bleeping normally rises to almost the same level as when testing the cable directly. Then get the person to hold hands with another and test the far hand of the second person. You get a high frequency bleep as before.

In fact, you can go through a chain of four or five people stretching over a distance of ten or twelve feet before the intensity of the bleep even begins to fall much below that of the initial basic cable test! We have performed this test with nearly twenty people and the current flowed almost unimpeded to the last person on the chain. Furthermore, the same effect is demonstrable by placing the tracer probe against the interior socket outlet of a TV aerial connected to nothing more than an arrangement of wires on the roof (a TV aerial) and the TV itself. The same is true of the visual display units (VDU's) used in conjunction with most computers and word processors, and indeed practically all domestic appliances are surrounded by an electrical field which fades into the general background field present in buildings due to their content of electrical equipment and cabling. You may have seen demonstrations of this effect on television presentations concerning the suspected health hazards of VDU operators. In fact a TV, even if switched off, but still connected to the mains electricity supply, is also a powerful emitter of electromagnetic radiation. Generally speaking, it is a good practice to switch off all electrical devices at their wall sockets, whenever possible, to prevent emissions from the cable and the device itself. So the old lady was right, 'I won't have that in my house, leaking all over the place', she is supposed to have said!

You may also notice that some individuals are better conductors than others – one individual will cause more of a damping of the bleep frequency than another. This is because, not only do electrical skin resistance and surface skin moisture content vary from person to person, but also because the body has an electrical capacitance, which varies. That is, the body stores the electrons which make up the flow of electricity. This storage of the electrons in metal objects on the body as well as in the bone and tissue structure can cause a reversal of the polarities or disharmony in the subtle energy fields. Metal objects include jewellery, buckles, fasteners, mattress springs while we sleep etc., and most importantly – tooth fillings. There have been reports of people who live near radio or TV transmitters actually producing recognisable radio broadcasts from their mouth! The metal acts as an aerial and a combination of the semi-conductive nature of the tooth fillings and body tissues, plus the acoustic resonance of the skull results in the emanation of sound.

Recent research on dental amalgams show that mercury as mercuric ions, can come into solution from tooth fillings due to differential electrical potentials being created in the mouth, in much the same way as a battery. The effect of induced currents in tooth fillings is also likely to enhance this effect. You can readily test for induced currents due to electric cabling or radio and TV broadcasting with a voltage tracer: the instrument will bleep at any metal or conductive object in close proximity to an electric cable – a wire coat-hanger, a metal-framed lampshade or any part of the human body... not just the hands! It would make an interesting survey to discover if electrical power and radio/TV broadcast engineers have higher than average mercury in their bodies.

I remember one girl who came to me for treatment, mainly because she had a tendency to give people an electric shock on personal contact. Being French, where kisses and handshakes are handed out in large numbers on a day to day basis, her problem was an embarrassment! On testing with a voltage tracer, I discovered that no current passed through her at all. That is, she was a very good capacitor. She stored all the electricity on her body and occasionally passed it on to others carrying less charge – a warm, wet kiss being an ideal contact for the transfer of electricity!

There was another interesting fact about her. When I asked her to remove all metal objects from her person prior to treatment, I discovered: four metal bracelets, two long metal earrings, three metal rings and just one big key on a twelve inch chain. She also told me that she was not wearing the brass medallion normally worn as a pendant on a chain. In other words, she was amplifying her own body's tendency to store electricity. Like an addict, she was drawn to the very thing causing her problem. I only saw her the one time, since she was on vacation in Cambridge and left soon after, but I did hear that the ringing in her ears, the other reason for her seeking treatment, had gone away and that wearing less metalwork on her person was also proving helpful to her general feeling of well-being.

During the exceptionally cold spell in the British Isles during February 1986, my wife and I started receiving discharge shocks when touching electrical switches, getting into vehicles and occasionally when touching other people. I also had a number of phone calls from people in various parts of the country experiencing the same phenomenon. One assumes that some aspect of the weather conditions was responsible and I mention it simply to point to the dynamic nature of the electromagnetic forces present in nature. Someone also suggested that the solar wind of sub-atomic particles responsible for the Aurora Borealis and other atmospheric electrical phenomena might have been affected by Haley's Comet, passing 'nearby' at the time, and creating an increase in the electrostatic field of the earth, resulting in a high level of atmospheric electrical activity.

Another young person that I met on a flight from Aberdeen to Edinburgh told me that she had a similar problem. On enquiry, I learnt that she worked as a switch-board operator at Aberdeen airport. I asked if she had any pains in her joints. 'Yes', was her surprised reply, as she wondered how I might have guessed it, 'In my right shoulder, sometimes so intense that I have to use my left hand on the switchboard . 'What about thunderstorms', I asked. 'Yes' was again the response. 'It can get worse at such times.' Pains in the joints seem to be connected with electrical imbalance in the body and conversely, magnetic treatments and foils are often of help in treating arthritis, rheumatism as well as sports and accident injuries. We will return to this topic on several occasions as the book progresses, but it seems that there is a biomagnetic and bioelectronic energy system within the body that is both organizational and information handling in its function. It acts somewhat as a subtle energy interface between the more vibrationally etheric or subtle states of matter and the sub-atomic, atomic and molecular levels of energy in our biophysical make-up, conveying the organizational patterning from within into outward manifestation.

The electromagnetic energy spectrum can be considered as follows:

10^{29}	10^{26}	10^{18}	$1^{16}0$	1.75×10^{14}	10^{14}	10^{12}	10^{10}–10^{4}	50–0
Cosmic Rays	Gamma Rays	X-Rays	Ultra Violet	Visible Light	Infra Red	Micro- waves Radar	Radio & TV	ELF

the proportions of this diagram being way out! Some of the frequencies in cycles per second (Hertz or Hz) are written above. 10^{10}, for example, means 1, followed by ten zeros and ELF means Extremely Low Frequency.

While studying this list, it is particularly interesting to note that most of the electromagnetic spectrum is already known to be injurious to health.

Other species have senses that detect other parts of this spectrum as well as magnetic fields. Owls and probably other night-flying predatory birds perceive the infra-red or heat emanations of their prey. Geese have been observed to be disoriented by ELF broadcasts. Brimstone butterflies and many other insects including honey bees are sensitive to ultra-violet light. In fact, when one brimstone butterfly looks at another brimstone butterfly (they are the big yellow ones that we in Europe see during autumn and spring), then they see patterns on what to us are simple yellow wings.

Bees are also sensitive to both the direction of polarization of light waves – their angle of vibration – as well as being magnetically sensitive to the earth's magnetic field. As von Frisch discovered many years ago, bees communicate the location of a source of food by performing a 'waggle dance' on the vertical surface of a honeycomb. The angle from the vertical indicates the angle to the sun at which the bees have to fly in order to find the food source. This angle is also corrected for wind direction and velocity. But if the earth's magnetic field within the hive is nullified by means of an external electric coil, then the angle of dance is also changed.

In fact, bees, pigeons, ducks, dolphins, butterflies, moles, tunafish, bacteria, turtles, crustacea and humans have all been found to contain magnetite crystals, Fe_3O_4, the naturally occuring lodestone of the ancient pilots. Some bacteria automatically swim towards a North pole and others towards a South pole. Some will seek a positive electrical potential, others will swim to a negative potential. In one particular species, at least, iron makes up 2% of its dry weight, with most of this being found as minute particles of magnetite, bound in membranes and arranged longitudinally, traversing the cell. This effectively becomes a magnet that automatically orientates the bacteria in the geomagnetic field.

In higher species there would apparently be some means of conveying the orientation of these magnetic crystals to the central nervous system and hence to the sensory awareness of the creature itself. Some magnetotactic bacteria have also been found living symbiotically in human blood where they are involved in the essential process of forming a clot, to stop bleeding.

The point is that other species are aware of energy fields and vibrations that we are not. A sensory experience is simply an ability to detect changes in energy patterns and there is absolutely no reason why all creatures should respond to the same energy vibrations and have the same senses. It means too, that living creatures are sensitive to electrical, electromagnetic and magnetic influences and that our inability to perceive these energies does not mean that they will not be modifying or interacting with our essential life functions and subtle energy systems.

An early 1985 article in the New Scientist, describes how the electrical charge on blood cells varies in health and disease. The work of Dr. Harold Saxton Burr on changes in the pure electrical potentials on and around the body's surface show a direct relationship to health, disease and rhythmic body function, and in the next chapter we discuss the work of Davis and Rawls in mapping these potentials and the use of this knowledge in therapy. Some modern hospital researchers are using electromagnetic and magnetic fields in their treatment of muscular injuries, as well as bone and joint problems, including rheumatism and arthritis, showing once again that the body is sensitive to low level external electrical and electromagnetic activity. We will return to this topic later in the book, what I want to emphasize here is that the body has electromagnetic energy fields which can be disturbed by environmental electromagnetism.

We are all aware of the harmful effects of certain parts of the electromagnetic spectrum. X-rays, microwave and ultra-violet are particularly well known, other aspects are not so well documented or easy to identify.

There is some evidence suggesting that the emanation of microwave ovens, for example, can cause health problems, including cataracts of the eye.

The case of the film set who were irradiated by radioactive fall-out when the wind changed direction during a U.S. Nevada Desert Atomic Explosion Test has become quite well-known. Now, fifteen to twenty years later, many of the cast and film crew are dying or have died of cancer, including John Wayne, Susan Hayward and Clark Gable. Similarly, with the ground zero engineers who were ordered into the area before it was contamination free.

Recent research in the U.K. has related a higher than average incidence of suicide and psychological disturbances amongst people living near high voltage electricity pylons, within their very high induction field. Along these lines, the village of Fishpond in Dorset has been the subject of much recent enquiry.

In both the U.K. and U.S.A., a number of studies have independently identified significantly increased incidences of leukaemia and other cancers amongst those living in close proximity (50 to 100 yards) to overhead power cables. Similar studies in those occupationally exposed to mains frequency electomagnetic fields identify a higher risk of leukaemia, as well as studies involving amateur radio operators in the U.S.A. and electrical power workers in New Zealand.

Andrew Marino, a biophysicist at the Veterans Administration Medical Centre in Syracuse, New York has shown in studies with both people and animals which simulated the electric and magnetic fields beneath high voltage cables, that intensities equivalent to those directly beneath power cables can cause a stunting of growth. Field strengths similar to those a hundred to two hundred yards away cause physiological effects such as changes in heart rate and blood chemistry, while levels experienced at distances of three to four hundred yards resulted in behavioural effects, such as a lowering of human reaction time.

There are many cases that can be quoted. The point is that this kind of electromagnetic pollution may not show up in serious illness for as long as fifteen to twenty years after the event. This has been observed on many occasions. Furthermore, it is very difficult to quantify the effect of continual bombardment by low intensity electromagnetic radiation such as TV and radio broadcasting and ordinary mains circuit emissions in domestic and commercial properties.

The small, picturesque town of Canonsburg in Pennsylvania housed a uranium extraction and processing factory, whose only customer from 1942 to 1957 was the United States Government. The uranium was used in the manufacture of atomic bombs. Sylvia Collier, in her Observer article of March 10th, 1985, writes: 'No one ever imagined that any harm could come from the familiar old factory. Local people would help themselves to sand and rubble lying around the site and cart it away to turn into patios, garden paths and blocks for building. A Government survey has now found 130 radioactive 'hot spots' all over town, including bedroom walls, tool sheds, doorsteps, bath tubs and children's sandpits.'

The baseball field where the youngsters used to play, now lies guarded behind a chain link fence along with eighteen adjacent acres in the heart of the country town. 'Yellow and purple signs bristle along the fence', writes Sylvia Collier, marked: 'No Entry, Radio-active Material.'

The U.S. Government insists that there is no health hazard despite the fact that many of the boys who played there, along with numerous other inhabitants, have died of cancer during their twenties. Mrs Janis Dunn, prompted by cancer in her family and the strange atmosphere surrounding the house she and her husband built next to the dump, conducted her own private survey in 1980. Knocking on forty-five doors, she discovered sixty-seven cases of cancer. In one street with fifty-nine people, she found twenty cancer cases.

The significance of the long time-lapse between exposure to low levels of radiation and its manifestation as disease or cancer can be readily understood. The body cells are in a constant state of reproduction of the new and destruction and re-absorption of the old. Some blood cells last for only a day, while brain cells are thought never to be replaced throughout a lifetime – there are simply a multitude of spare brain cells that replace those that die, these being replaced by fatty cells. Other cells have a lifetime of months or years. It is said, for example, that when you meet someone after a period of six months, not one cell on his face will be the same as on your previous meeting.

The mechanisms by which cells proliferate, producing identical copies of themselves, are inherent in both the long protein molecules within the cell nucleus, the chromosomes, as well as in the subtle energy blueprints or patterns which precipitate or manifest at the molecular, chromosomal level. In simplified language, these controlling proteins and their subtle counterpart act as a mold, a pattern or a template, for the next generation of cells. They simply copy themselves. The protein molecules are long and complex. It is the inter-relationships of atoms within the molecules, the spatial and vibrational arrangement of the energy patterns, that give rise to physical characteristics (black hair, blue eyes, etc.), as well as to specific control of physiological function.

From a karmic point of view, the energy patterns that give rise to our destiny are etched into the fabric of our antashkarans, our physical mind. From here they manifest outwardly through the genetic control points within the cellular nucleus as well as in all other aspects of our inner and so-called outer life. It is therefore quite true to say that we have created our own environment as well as all the events that come our way – great or small. We are co-creators of the world we live in. This is why the things which happen to us so often reflect our inner attitudes and personality. Conversely, we are also born with a certain personality or nature which predisposes us to get involved in those situations to which we are destined.

Returning, however, to our discussion of subtle, molecular and genetic patterns. Electromagnetic radiation and radioactive particle emissions are able to disharmonize or even break up these subtle energy and protein patterns. The proteins may rejoin themselves correctly, they may die or they may rejoin in a new pattern, with potentially destructive qualities. If only a small number of cells are so damaged, it may take fifteen to twenty years before the children of these cells and their progeny represent a large enough proportion of the total cell population to pose a threat to the health of the individual. Hence, the long time delays between exposure to radiation and the manifestation of ill-health.

Furthermore, the disturbances in the subtle energy field may remain after even low intensity exposure, perhaps at an information storage level, to cause disease at a later stage of life when natural resistance is lower.

The body, of course, has its own way of dealing with strangers, which can in any event, occur naturally and be dealt with naturally. The stronger the individual's subtle energy fields and degree of health, the more his ability to cope with dis-ease or dis-harmony.

Cancerous cells may also develop the bad habit of reproducing continuously. Most cells divide and pause. Malignant cancerous cells show no such inhibitions and thus they can gain control.

Anything therefore, which disharmonizes the subtle energy patterns or the molecular structure of the chromosomal proteins can be carcinogenic. Hence, there are also chemicals and viruses which can cause cancer.

There have recently been a number of reports indicating a statistically significant proportion of miscarriages and embryonic deformities amongst expectant mothers working on VDU's – computers and word processors etc.

Embryo deformities can be the result of chromosomal damage. Chromosomal damage can be caused by electro-magnetic radiation. VDU's (and TV's) emit electromagnetic radiation. As we described above, chromosomal damage becomes most rapidly apparent in cells which are dividing rapidly. Embryonic cells are naturally dividing rapidly – this is what constitutes their growth and the more subtle organizational, information-encoded, subtle blueprints are naturally operating at high 'capacity' during embryological development. Therefore, small doses of radiation will have greater damaging effect on embryos over a short period of time, than on adults. Moreover, the total structure of the organism is derived from the chromosomes, so any embryonic, chromosomal damage will also be liable to cause deformities. And finally, one cause of miscarriage is deformity – the body's natural mechanisms detect problems and the foetus is aborted. The effect of VDU's on expectant mothers is therefore quite readily understandable.

Recent studies of only three to five years on the effects of irradiating foods with X-rays and gamma rays for the purposes of sterilization, giving them longer shelf-life, before sale to the public, is therefore – in the light of the above – just not long enough. The food, they say, is left with 'minimal' induced radioactivity and the supposedly positive factor (for the suppliers) that – for example – potatoes don't sprout after such irradiation, only goes to show that the all important life energy of the potato is thoroughly destroyed. If such radiation destroys bacteria and viruses, then you can be sure that our 'fresh' fruit and vegetables will also have been denatured when treated in this manner. The subject of food irradiation is discussed more fully in my book, *Radiation*.

Moreover, the effects of such high energy, even if low intensity, destructive irradiation on the polarities and harmony within subtle energy fields can only be negative. Similarly, with microwave cookers. The molecular structure, as well as the subtle energy aspects, are bound to be disturbed. It is simply industrial and economic greed, as well as ignorance, that provides the impetus for glossing over the obvious dangers.

The rapid turnover of blood cells also relates to one of

the more common forms of cancer – leukaemia – an uncontrolled proliferation of the white blood cells. White blood cells are produced by the spleen and it is well known that the subtle counterpart of the spleen is a major centre or chakra for the assimilation and distribution of subtle energies throughout the body. So one can readily understand part of the reason why microwaves, electric fields and nuclear radiation all affect this centre, resulting in leukaemia. The spleen and the white blood cells are also an important part of the immune system which when disturbed in its subtle aspects would result in an imbalance and hyperactivity of the spleen, again leading towards a high white cell count.

There are many parallels, too, in other areas of environmental pollution. DDT, for example, was heralded as a boon to pest control. It was later found to be harmful to human health and the recommended quantities to be used by farmers were drastically reduced. Later on, as it became evident that DDT is both stored in the body over long periods, is poisonous and carcinogenic and non-biodegradable so that it remains in the soil year after year – it became a 'non-recommended' (not illegal) chemical. Recent evidence however, published by the Sunday Times, shows that one third of all our food is contaminated by DDT and other lethal chemicals. Either farmers are still using DDT and/or the DDT used many years ago and remaining in the soil is still causing problems. DDT and similar chemicals are still being used by developing world countries which supply many foodstuffs to our country.

Similarly, what is discounted today as unharmful electromagnetic radiation may, in the light of further evidence, prove to have highly injurious effects on our long-term health and well-being. It would be interesting to have accurate statistics on the relationship between the high incidence of cancer and heart disease and the build up in usage over the last three decades of electrical appliances, computer, VDU and electronic equipment and especially TV and radio signal broadcasting and receiving. Workers in the field of energy balancing can relate reversals and disturbances in these subtle centres to electromagnetic bombardment. This is evidence enough for them, though it may not satisfy the more conventional and conservative mind.

In this respect, it is worth mentioning a theory that I have heard put forward by Dr. Yao of California. Therapists who understand the workings of the chakras or major spinal subtle energy centres in the body are aware that they are functionally associated with the major endocrine glands. Hormones are key chemical triggers, energy vibrations with far reaching effects in both our emotional and mental, as well as physical energy patterns. Now because electromagnetic energy is closely related to more subtle energies, electromagnetic pollution can cause subtle energy disharmonies in these major chakras.

Dr. Yao's work relates a specific subtle polarity to chakras which is opposite in men and women. The sex centre, for example, is negative or receptive in woman and positive in a man. This difference is responsible for the production of oestrogen and progesterone in the female and testosterone in the male. All these three hormones are, by the way, very similar in biochemical structure and can be transmuted by the body, one into another, i.e. their vibrational 'being' is similar. They are however partially responsible for the maintenance of the dissimilar secondary sexual characteristics, including sexual proclivities and feelings, psychology and body hair etc.

If, therefore, the vibration within the sacral chakra is disturbed and its polarity reversed, due to electromagnetic or any other influences, then there is a likelihood of excess production of the wrong hormone as a direct biochemical reflection of the reversed vibrations or polarity.

The net result is a homosexual tendency which may or may not be expressed, depending upon its degree as well as other factors both within the individual and his or her environment. The increasing incidence of unisex social behaviour, of homosexuality and a merging of secondary sexual characteristics in urban environments where, electromagnetic pollution is high and the stabilizing effects of the earth's natural magnetic and electrostatic fields are absent, can perhaps be partially explained therefore, by electromagnetic disharmonizing of the body chakras. This would make an interesting and beneficial research project. In fact, back in 1969 Dr. Karel M. Marha, Institute of Industrial Hygiene and Occupational Diseases, Praha, in Czechoslovakia published reports of complaints amongst electrical power workers that included memory and hearing losses and headaches, as well as disturbances to menstrual cycles and sexual potency.

It is possible, too, that the AIDS virus has its source in vibrational disharmony, manifesting ultimately as a reproducing complex molecule or virus and finding a home for growth in those people already containing the causal or resonant vibration. This theory would explain why AIDS is a 'new disease' in our western culture (due to the new environmental pollution), why it is particularly effective in striking homosexuals, (reversed, disharmonized polarities in tune with the AIDS vibration) and why only a small proportion of people with the virus show symptoms (they don't have the sympathetic, disharmonized vibration in them).

Bio-Entrainment

The bio-energy, subtle force field or aura of the body is also affected by sympathetic resonance with similar force fields. This partly explains, for example, why husband and wife who have lived together for many years can take on very similar features in both physical appearance, as well as in mental and emotional attitudes. They are living within each other's aura and their vibrations become attuned to each other. This will occur whether or not they are a harmonious couple, though one would expect mental and emotional harmony to enhance the merging process.

We are also affected by the presence of other people on a day to day basis. Note also how moods can take over an entire crowd or room full of people. We talk, too, of atmospheres – good or bad – that build up amongst groups of people. We also find that certain places, homes or individual rooms have 'good' or 'bad' vibrations and affect us accordingly.

When this effect is long term, it creates a habit in our body, known as 'bio-entrainment', a form of subtle energy resonance, and while we may be happy to be uplifted by good vibrations, we would prefer to avoid the drag of the negative.

The experience of the majority of users of the bio-crystal Pulsor® devices mentioned in the next chapter is that they amplify the body's natural aura, providing a strong, protective force field in which one is more able to influence others than have them influence us. When in places with a negative atmosphere, users report feeling cocooned and cushioned against its potential effect on them.

Entrainment of brain and body functions can also occur from electromagnetic radiation. The heart, brain and muscles all emit signals from less than one cycle per second to over a hundred thousand cycles per second. These signals form the basis of electrocardiograms and electroencephalograms. Amidst all this electrical activity, four predominant brain wave patterns can be identified:

Delta	0.5 to 3Hz	Deep sleep, higher states of consciousness
Theta	4 to 7Hz	Reverie, dream states
Alpha	8 to 13Hz	Passive, blank, relaxed, meditation
Beta	14 to 30Hz	Thinking, active mind and/or body

ELF (extremely low frequency) electromagnetic emissions at these frequencies are thus likely to be psychoactive. That is, they can affect your mood. It is said that the USSR and the USA have both developed and use such weapons. They call it 'world mood manipulation' and 'psychotronic warfare'.

A recent BBC TV documentary revealed that the Soviet Union has built the three largest broadcasting stations ever designed. From these stations are broadcast a pulsed electromagnetic signal that is receivable as a click on a shortwave radio. This is the most powerful electromagnetic signal ever broadcast. The given code name is 'Woodpecker' and both the U.S.A. and Europe – but not the U.S.S.R. – are targets for this emission. The U.S.A. have responded by building a similar transmitter, the signals from which are bounced off the ionosphere, but the Soviet Union now have many years research behind them on psycho-active, electromagnetic frequencies.

The brain also has a weak magnetic field associated with it. Davis and Rawls, back in the 1960's and 1970's were amongst the first to point out that the powerful cobalt samarian magnets used in telephones will detrimentally affect the fuctioning of your brain whenever you hold the earpiece close to your head. Many people have commented upon the energy drain experienced by using the telephone. No doubt, this can also be due to receiving an earful of rubbish from somebody, but this is only infrequently the case! Similarly, electric hair dryers and shavers produce electromagnetic fields and radiation which are bound to interact with brainwave patterns and brain function.

In fact, Dr. Ross Adey, when at the Brain Research Institute at UCLA in 1973, discovered that exposure of monkeys to electromagnetic radiation of frequencies surrounding us at all times, resulted in behavioural changes and a distortion in their sense of time. Adey and many other scientists believe that the bodily rhythms that govern our cyclic and other activities – waking, sleeping and many more subtle processes – are regulated by entrainment to the earth's natural magnetic and electrostatic fields.

In the presence of ambient and artificial electromangnetic fields, it seems likely that we respond by adjusting our rhythms to that of the electronic 'smog.' As a result, the body, mind and emotional complex undergo stress and natural processes break down, leaving us prone to disease patterns to which we would have otherwise remained immune. In Western countries, it is only since the 1970's that any extensive research has been undertaken, but in Russia and Eastern Europe, hundreds of experiments have shown that electromagnetic fields may cause a host of health problems, including blood disorders, hypertension, heart attacks, headaches, sexual disfunction, drowsiness and nervous exhaustion. The book: *Electromagnetic Fields and Life* by A.S. Presman from the Department of Biophysics, Moscow University, describes in detail many such experiments. It was first published in Russian in 1968 and translated into English in 1970.

As a result of their experimentation, the Soviet Union have strict rules over the amount and duration of emission from radio transmitters and radars that a person can safely absorb. The West has only an informal, non-legal guideline set in 1966 by the U.S. American Standards Institute. The Soviet criteria are one thousand times tougher than this for workers and ten thousand times more for the general public. Clearly, the Russians believe that even small doses of electromagnetic smog, over time, can do great harm.

In his January 1980 article in the U.S. edition of *The Readers Digest*, Lowell Ponte from whom the above information was quoted, graphically describes the well-known tale of Russian microwave irradiation of the U.S. Embassy in Moscow. In 1962, he says, the CIA discovered that the Soviets were beaming microwaves into the U.S. embassy in Moscow, deliberately aimed at the U.S. ambassador's office from two buildings across the street. It was .002 of the intensity that the American guideline called dangerous.

The CIA set up experiments to duplicate the irradiation on monkeys and within three weeks there were adverse effects on the animals' nervous and immune systems.

Embassy officials, however were not informed of the irradiation. Instead they were asked to give blood samples to 'test for a disease in Moscow's water'. These tests revealed that about a third had a white blood cell count almost fifty percent higher than normal – often a symptom of severe infection and also a characteristic of leukaemia.

In 1976, the U.S. State Department declared the Moscow embassy an 'unhealthful post', and metal window screens were put up to shield against the microwave beams. But this was fourteen years after their discovery. Today, those former embassy personnel exhibit a higher rate of cancer than the American average, and two U.S. ambassadors in Moscow subjected to this radiation have died of cancer.

We relate these incidents concerning the 'superpowers', not in any political spirit or wish to create divisions amongst our fellow humans, but simply because they highlight certain problem areas. Some of these incidents sound almost unbelievable, yet so does the creation of nuclear devices designed to destroy life completely for the sake of political or economic ideals. Why do humans inflict such suffering on themselves?

Addiction to Electromagnetic Radiation – Computer & Video Junkies

Talking with people and observing the compelling and obsessive behaviour of those 'hooked' on computers and television, one cannot help wondering if, in fact, such strong electromagnetic radiations are habit forming in the manner of a drug – i.e. bio-entrainment. The body gets used to having its polarities reversed or its energies disharmonized and craves a continuance of the process. Many people have told me, quite independently, that watching television, even for just a short while, leaves them with a feeling of energy depletion – and yet they find it difficult to break the habit or even to switch it off. Feeling tired all the time is a common symptom of computer junkies and TV addicts. It is also a symptom of reversed polarities and disharmonized subtle energy. The addiction cannot be explained simply as 'just psychological', though even with psychological aspects there has to be an energy pathway linking the physical to the emotional and mental. The frequent comment from many of the 'older generation' that modern young people seem unable to have the stamina to do a good day's work may have a basis in this reality. The 'wired-up' nature of computer and video games junkies is a characteristic of their type and of many folk working continually with electronic equipment; Pulsor treatment usually revealing polarity reversals. I have had a number of such individuals express to me that after Pulsor® treatment, they have felt good in a way not experienced for a long time, if ever. In the U.S.A., a survey has shown that there is a percentage of the current young generation, classifiable as computer junkies, who have severe communication and social problems. It is imperative that these problems are recognised, taken seriously, made public and solutions found.

The Earth's Magnetism and Subtle Energy Fields

Our earth itself is surrounded and permeated by its own magnetic, electrostatic, gravitational and more subtle energy fields. These fields react with similar levels of energy within the body for good or ill. Thus we find areas of good atmosphere and bad atmosphere – places, sometimes quite localized, which have a history of poor health or failing enterprises and others where the reverse is true.

We go into this in more detail in chapters seven and eight, but the point to be brought out here is that subtle energy polarities and harmony are affected directly by these energies.

Thus the disorientation aspects of jet lag and some kinds of motion sickness are also related to subtle energy field disharmonies caused by the frequent crossing of the magnetic field of the earth, one feels jangled. This is why an east-west journey is worse in effect than north-south. There is also evidence to suggest that air-line pilots and hostesses suffer premature aging. It also explains, too, why those with a weak, easily influenced or sensitive subtle energy system are more readily 'shattered' by jet lag. Again, we have found that carrying bio-crystals on one's person holds the subtle energies in balance and mitigates much of the effect of crossing the earth's magnetic field.

Similarly, living over underground water or at intersections of earth energy networks, create a negative vibration which can cause subtle energy disharmonies amongst those dwelling there.

CHAPTER 5

Polarity Balancing Therapies

In the previous chapter, we discussed subtle energy harmony and polarity. This chapter is devoted to discussing some of the therapies that work through the balancing of polarities, clearing energy blockages and generally creating harmony within the energy flow patterns. This is in addition to the healthful flow of energy attributable to a harmonious and well-balanced lifestyle. We restrict ourselves to just three of those therapies that specifically think in terms of polarity as the essential basis of energy flow, and which are also the result of *western* research and synthesis. I have also had the good luck to be personally associated with two of these three techniques. Acupuncture, acupressure, Ta'i Ch'i, Hatha Yoga, radionics and other techniques that balance subtle energy flow patterns have been described specifically by experts of those disciplines and are already more widely known.

Dr. Stone's Polarity Therapy

Dr. Randolf Stone died in India, at the age of 91, in the year of 1981. For the last thirty or forty years of his life, he had been an initiate of a mystic adept of the highest order, Maharaj Sawan Singh Ji. Originally a chiropractor by training, Dr. Stone became steeped in the eastern wisdom and through his understanding of the inner structure of the universe and of the gunas described both in the Hindu literature and by his own guru, he came to define techniques for balancing the energy flow in human beings.

Dr. Stone was a strong and forthright personality whom I had the good fortune to meet in India on a number of occasions during the late 1960's. Those who were close to him at his death said that he died radiant and peaceful, happy that his life's term of karma had been completed. He practised and taught his Polarity Therapy in both California and India with great success, leaving behind voluminous writings and some well-trained professional therapists and teachers of his work. This work is continued today in many countries of the world.

Dr. Stone summarizes his philosophy of health and disease in his introductory book: *Health Building – The Conscious Art of Living Well*, first published in 1962 and now available in an American edition (see bibliography).

He describes something of his background when he says:

'For more than 45 years, I have been making research into energy fields in their relation to the healing art. Only I started with the life principle in the centre and worked outward in its application. I studied most of the ancient concepts of life and their approach to the life in man as an energy radiation principle in Nature in relation to the unit of life in man. It was called odic fluid, mesmerism, animal magnetism, and many other names. Man's constitution in the finer energy fields of mind, emotions, electromagnetic light waves, radiations and their effect on the chemistry in the cell as polarity energy of attraction and repulsion, is the reality behind these names.

'All cells are bipolar or they could not act and funtion. The law of polarity – of positive, negative and neuter energy – rules all matter as the principle of the three gunas from the (universal) mind downward. Attraction and repulsion is the manifestation of life, as in the sex-polarity of male and female through all creation of vegetation, animals and humans. Even metals have their positive and negative polarity, like the values of gold and silver which attract the sun and moon energies and are fine conductors for electronic construction. Much silver is being used for it nowadays.

'In this research, I have stumbled onto a science which blends the old concept of energies in the constitution of man and have linked it with the scientific research in space as the magnetosphere and electromagnetic lines of force in man's constitution. In my books and courses for doctors, I had drawings made which outline this in detail in relationship to the anatomy and physiology of the body. This relationship is the art of Polarity Therapy, based on the primary mind pattern energy in the brain which is duplicated in every oval[1]of the body as the five bases for sensory perception and motor function by which we live and act. Near as it is to us, nevertheless it is a lost art called the Spagyric Art by the great medieval doctor, Paracelsus von Hoenheim. He was taught its secrets in Arabia and in other parts of the then travelled world, even among shepherds and gypsies who lived near the grass roots of life with some strange traditions and secrets from the past. It became a lost art again after the great doctor passed on in Salzburg, Austria, on September 24, 1541.

'His great contribution was the use of the electromagnetic energy waves to human chemistry. His research and knowledge in chemistry gave a great boost to that science, but the real secret of the electromagnetic energy connection to chemistry was lost to the world. Only chemistry in its grosser form survived and the world benefitted by it.

'*Polarity Therapy* is the name I gave to this art of correspondences of body spaces and functions, through attraction and repulsion of electromagnetic energy waves as the root of the five senses – sensory and motor – functioning in the body. Linking it with the cerebrospinal fluid radiation and circulation brought it into the realm of physiology and through the brain, the spinal cord and nerves and its meningeal coverings, made it a tangible asset in research and in the practice of the Healing Art. Polarity Therapy provides a definite location for the electromagnetic fields and their directive life-giving energy in man, which can be used as a definite art in therapeutics.

'When we are ill,' he writes, 'and have pains, we think that it is the body which hurts and is sick, when in reality it is the life-breath or Prana Currents in the body (which operate it and sustain it), which are out of balance and coordination in their polarity function of attraction and repulsion. This negative and positive action throughout the system is the factor which makes each cell contract and expand in its process of life: to take in nourishment – of solids, liquids, gases, warmth or energy – use it, and discard the waste products and gases and to radiate the heat (or caloric) energy for use and distribution.

[1]Dr. Stone refers here to the five ovals of the torso: the head, the neck, the chest, the abdomen and the pelvis.

'This seems a new idea or concept, because we approach and explain it from the modern basis of energy radiation, conduction and absorption, like electronic engineers would in their atomic research. This energy approach is prior to chemistry and mechanics. Energy in its threefold action of positive (+), negative (–), and neuter (0) polarity is prior to chemistry which deals with particles of matter and their chemical affinity – or antipathy – and which can result in new combinations.'

Scientists generally, as Dr. Stone also points out, are so involved with the ramifications of activity and energy interchange in chemistry, engineering, biology, medicine, physics and so on, that the significance of the basic polarity or duality in nature, underlying all these energy inter-changes, is altogether ignored. It is only relatively few scientists – though an increasing number – who appreciate the beauty and reality of the simplicity inherent in this understanding and realize the real nature of the scientific idiom itself as an approach to understanding the cosmos. It is, after all, just an idiom – not an absolute verity.

Matter, or *maya*, is too powerful an illusion for us to withstand. That which is manifest to our senses and in-strumentation appears so *real* that the deeper layers of life are easily ignored. If we approach life in a superficial manner and attempt to solve its problems sympto-matically, then this is automatically reflected in our ap-proach to science and medicine. The deeper the man, the deeper his science. And this is true on an individual, as well as sociological and disciplinary level.

According to Dr. Stone, the life energy in both subtle and electromagnetic form has its seat in the brain and spinal cord as a highly energetic, intense and vibrating subtle essence. Through the positive and negative polari-ties of this field, appearing at the physical level as electro-magnetic energy, the vital life energy is driven throughout the otherwise dead matter of the body infusing it with the life principle. All pain, he says, is due to obstructions in this flow at molecular, electromagnetic and more subtle energy levels. Harmonize and balance the polarities – the motor or driving force of the life energy – and health is restored, whilst the pain automatically disappears from the consciousness. Supress the symptoms and the underlying imbalance will automatically manifest itself in some other, perhaps more imbalanced and serious, way.

Health comes by removing all obstructions between the inner life force and the outer physical body. Then the source of all love, life and energy is allowed to flow unimpeded creating health, success and happiness. God runs a beauty parlour, it is said, and certainly He could run a health parlour, too, if His life energy and being is allowed to infuse our own, straightening out all the distorted, blocked, stagnant and confused energy pathways of our mental-emotional-physical complex.

With this point of understanding, Dr. Stone, therefore underlines the importance of a healthy mind and emotional structure as formulators of positive and negative energy flow and balanced biochemistry. Negative thoughts and emotions are blockages in the free flow of life energy and manifest ultimately as degenerative conditions. The seeker of health must develop a balanced and positive attitude and a feeling of being at one with themselves, with others and with nature.

Emotion manifests itself rapidly as biochemistry. The angry and disturbed person, for example, develops an acid system, a preponderance of the positively charged H^+ ion. Their thought and emotional patterns are so blocked that they become set like a continuous gramophone record playing in the higher energy fields, ultimately manifesting themselves as acidic digestive problems with ulcers, as rheumatism and arthritic stagnation and crystallization, as hardening of the arteries and heart problems.

The acidic system attracts to itself the very foods that cause an increase in acidity. Like the drug addict unable to resist the drug, the hyperactive, but rigid, intolerant and prejudiced acidic nature seeks tension, coffee, sweet, starchy and fatty foods, alcohol and the like. An influx of balanced life energy from within is the only remedy that will stem the inevitable decline, backed up with counselling or education and a change of dietary and living patterns. To treat an ulcer or a heart complaint with a drug is so superficial, it is negligent in terms of human observation, as well as available treatment. It is simply papering over the cracks.

Negative mental attitudes attract negative energy at all

levels, whilst positive attitudes engender the absorption of positive energy from the etheric and subtle fields that surround us, both within and without. We become that upon which we consciously or unconsciously contemplate. 'We make the bed we lie on. We build the house we live in,' says Dr. Stone.

Dr. Stone's writings contain a beautiful expression of polarity principles as applied to basic health. The greatest natural healers have all pursued their work as might an artist or poet, but with a firm foundation of science and knowledge. They are children of nature, a gift to mankind to maintain the balance of health. No doubt you will see in it many ideas and concepts expressed in a slightly different manner or idiom to my own, but containing the same essential observations and thinking.

In poetic and mystic mood, Dr. Stone again writes: 'Life is the expression of love in sound waves and energy currents, throughout the creation and in man. Love is light, which crystallizes as beauty in the spectrum, becomes color and gases as it is reduced in its speed of vibration and also forms the beautiful colors in the buds, the flowers, and the fruits. It precipitates as the delicate pink color in the lacework of tissues in the human form. Everywhere is seen the expression of love and beauty as art and design patterns. Concentrated waves form electromagnetic fields, build the cells and govern them by attraction and repulsion. The three gunas are everywhere as the attributes of matter and motion, as positive (+), negative (−), and neuter (0). Everywhere is life in motion, and in sound effects such as speech, the songs of birds, and the lowing of beasts or their roar of life's expression. There is music everywhere as plus and minus tones, without and within, if we can but hear it and see it in love and understanding of the Creator's Grace and Being. He is the essence of all life and beauty everywhere. With this keynote of understanding, life flows like a river with its natural expression as health.'

Dr. Stone often talks of positive and negative 'space particles', and is, I believe, referring to the subtle akash or etheric element, sometimes referred to as 'space' or 'vacuum.' The different living organisms have varying proportions of the five elements in their make up. Man being the only species with all five interacting together. It is this element that gives us our capacity for rational (and also irrational) thought. Since this is a vibrating energy field like everything else, Dr. Stone is thinking of 'particles' or concentrations of this energy that we attract to make up our thoughts – positive or negative – thus influencing our health and well-being at all levels.

Dr. Stone's usage of the term electromagnetic waves or electromagnetic light waves also goes beyond the normal scientific meaning of the term and includes the higher more subtle energies of which electromagnetic energy is the crystallization at lower physical levels. To inner vision, these currents in the body and the universe are indeed seen as a finer or primal essence of light, an aura, bathing the denser material of which they are the blueprint.

This is particularly clear, for example, when he talks of the 'electromagnetic' energy of life flowing from the great astral powerhouse of the Thousand Petalled Lotus. Clearly this is not the same energy as the electromagnetic spectrum which includes radio broadcast signals, light and X-rays.

Health is a state of balance, of neutral polarity, in which the positive and the negative are in balance, in a harmonious flow of life energy from within, expressed outwardly in balanced cellular and biochemical activity. The inner source is infinite in supply, it is a self-sustaining and complete system. 'Life then flows unconscious of itself in an exuberant expression as in childhood,' says the good doctor. This is the mystic tree of life that sustains the body through the flow of inner energy into the brain, the spinal cord and the body's subtle and gross energy transferring and transforming systems.

It is the principles of polarity, too, that permit our life energies to interchange with the energies of the cosmos. No energy interchange is passive, it is always interactive. When light falls on our body and is reflected, this is no static occurrence, but an interaction of electromagnetic energy with the molecules, atoms, electrical and other forces that comprise the material of which our gross bodies are made. This interaction is how blind people learn to feel colours or how people can know when they are in the vicinity of an electric field.

Dr. Stone's understanding resulted in a most detailed therapy in which diet, nutrition, lifestyle, exercise, counselling, hot and cold water therapy, sunbaths, special massage and polarity manipulation techniques, ways of balancing and augmenting energy flow and much more besides are all synthesized into one harmonious whole. Dr. Stone was superlatively practical in his approach. He was physically powerful, too. At the age of 78, I can well remember my amazement at seeing a heavy, spring-closed swing door fly open at the extension of the fingers of just one hand.

This underlying presence or absence of harmonious, balanced and vital life energy – or its blockage – explains why the same therapy applied to different people will have different effects and why a therapy may not always work. If the source of the trouble remains, then no amount of even natural and wholistic solutions will create a cure.

An over-concentration of acid, H^+, says Dr. Stone and many other natural physicians, is the source of cellular and biochemical hyperfunction and over-activity. An expression of the rajas or active guna, it causes redness, inflammation, swelling, heat and fever. These are also attributes of the fire element, an imbalance in which causes acute diseases that are self-limiting and are a part of nature's way of restoring balance and life, much as a fever can be cleansing and remedial when approached with understanding and not suppressed with drugs.

Over-alkalinity, OH^-, results in coldness, constriction, depression and dehydration. This is the source of all chronic conditions, an expression of the tamas guna. Again, there is an imbalance of polarity leading to constrictive illness and limited cellular function.

Pure water, H_2O, is the neutral pole between the two. H^+ and OH^- combine to form H_2O and we return to this topic shortly when discussing the effects of north and south magnetic poles on living organisms.

But it is always the flow of vital, inner energy that does the healing, at any level. This is why Chinese herbalism is specific about the yin (negative, female) and yang (positive, male) properties of the herbs used in their materia medica. Some herbs are therefore more suitable for some individuals than others, depending upon the yin and yang qualities of the patient. Organs, too, are seen as yin and yang, according to their role in total body function. The intestines are active, fiery and yang, for example, while the heart and lungs are nourishing, receptive and yin.

Dr. Stone had studied conventional, ayurvedic and natural medicine, chiropractic, acupuncture and much more. He had also, no doubt, read Rudolf Steiner and Alice Bailey on the more subtle aspects of healing, and his work has the hallmark of a great synthesizer and innovator. His charts of energy flow patterns and polarities in the body, as well as his work on the reflex manner in which energy is reflected through centres in the body, are extensive and often complex – the mind-emotion-body complex is, after all, a maze of interconnecting polarities and energy patterns. His method of treatment, however, was basically simple and involved the use of the natural polarities of the hands and the body. The atom and the cell are both bipolar, he says, with positive and negative charges in balance, dancing around and connected to a nucleus or neutral pole. This is indeed borne out by modern biochemistry which is aware of the negative charge on the cell membrane, the neutral cytoplasm and the positively charged nucleus.

Polarity therapy perceives the body somewhat in the nature of a magnified cell, an expansion of the balanced, neutral, life-force which has its seat in the brain and cerebrospinal fluid. The central axis of the human body is therefore neutral, while the right hand side of the body and head are positive, holding a positive electrical potential and radiating positive energy currents. The left side is negative – the reverse.

With a knowledge of this natural polarity, it becomes possible for every human being to balance their own energies and those of others and to relieve pain and discomfort.

An excess of *positive* sun-energy results in over-activity, inflammation and pain, as we have described. Placing the cooling, moon-energy of the *left palm* over such an area automatically results in soothing, refreshing and healing. For states of spasm, congestion or stagnation the activity-inducing *right palm* is required to bring life to torpid tissues.

All polarity healing takes place from side to side, from front to back, or from above to below and the healing power lies in the hands of every human being, though it is also true that some have a greater healing gift than others. Moreover, it is necessary for the one giving the treatment to be well-balanced for there will clearly be a transfer of energy from the therapist to the patient and vice-versa.

In practical terms, this means – to give a simple example – that if you have a pain towards the front on the body, then you should place your left hand over it, with your right hand at the same level aroud the back, to create a flow of energy through the imbalanced area. Similarly, for a headache you can put your left hand over the painful area and the right hand opposite it.

Pains in the spine can be treated with the palm of the left hand or with the hand doubled up into a fist, so that pressure or massage is also applied to the painful area. By lying on the left hand and by placing the right hand opposite to it, on the front of the body and lying in this way for ten or fifteen minutes (assuming that it does not require severe contortions!), then relief can often be gained, as the electromagnetic and subtle currents and fields are amplified and harmonized.

Similarly, it is polarity principles which underlie the age-old use of hot and cold water compresses. Heat draws positive energy and activity to an area – blood flow is brought to the surface capilliaries and nutrients brought to the tissues. Cold compresses relax and soothe an area, driving blood deeper into the tissues. However, the use of thermal energy is not so fundamental as the use of the left and right hands themselves, though under certain circumstances – ankle-sprains, for example – it is most appropriate and used widely by physiotherapists.

Hand movements and stroking also have soothing (left hand) or stimulating (right hand) effects as the energy of the therapist interacts with that of the patient. Similarly, downward stroking from the head to the feet is soothing – being in the direction of energy flow – whilst upward stroking, against the energy flow, has a stimulating effect. Both hands can be used for this since it is the direction of movement which determines the polarity. Furthermore, it is not necessary for the hands of the therapist to touch the patient, since the energy field of our body extends to some distance around ourselves.

Hand movements and stroking, of course, have psychologically energizing aspects, too, in terms of emotional nourishment, and recent studies in maternal habits have shown that those babies who are fondled and stroked thrive, gain weight and are generally more full of life than those who are neglected and left unattended. And in general, breast-fed and warmly reared children are healthier both emotionally and physically in later life.

Dr. Stone's understanding of diet and nutrition was once again based on the polarity of acid and alkaline, heating and cooling, yin and yang, energizing and soothing. Acid and alkaline foods, he said, should not be eaten together because they react upon each other causing fermentation and souring in the digestive tract. Citrus fruits and starches or cereals, for example, should not be eaten at the same meal, whilst sweet fruits and juices – raisins, dates, prunes, figs etc., combine well together and with cereals.

Conversely, proteins and acid foods, which both require an acid medium for their digestion, make suitable combinants.

This simple observation of acid and alkaline combinations can be readily seen in any school room chemistry class. The admixture of two acids will not normally result in an energetic reaction, while the mixing of acid and alkali reaches a stable, balanced state, with the formation of water, but often with the release of heat and general molecular agitation and rearrangement.

Dr. Stone also found the airy quality of citrus fruits of great nutritional benefit. In addition to aiding the digestion of protein foods, their high levels of calcium and phosporous actually result in an alkaline correction of overly acid systems, also supplying nutrition to the nervous and circulatory systems, as well as structural material for bones and teeth.

In these brief paragraphs, I have described just a few of the simpler methods devised by Dr. Stone over the course of half a century of study, research, practice and experimentation. His energy flow charts take into account the differing functions and polarities of all the bodily organs and systems, as well as incorporating the polarity principles inherent in the flow of the five elements or states of matter in the body and their major fields of function. His writings are full of insights into the manner of our human functioning and are well worth study.

Magnetism, Electrical Polarities and the Work of Davis and Rawls

Of all the forces in nature known to conventional science, those of magnetism and electricity are more understood and defined by the principles of polarity than any other. The entire fabric of their activity is clearly identifiable as action and force due to positive and negative charges, north and south poles.

Dr. H.S. Burr, as we have mentioned, was probably the first to correlate the activities of electrical potentials in the body with its general health and well-being. But, while Burr was not a student or seeker of higher and inner realities and he missed the real significance of his own work, Dr. Stone evolved his system from a combination of understanding universal principles and his empirical experience as a doctor. Dr. Stone worked from within out and from without in, to reach his results, Dr. Burr seems to have worked purely from without, in the manner of a open-minded, but conventional scientist.

The work of Davis and Rawls[1] represents an intermediate stage between the two approaches. They were both scientists, with their own private laboratory in which they conducted many thousands of experiments on the effects of magnetism and the natural electrical polarities that surround the body. They were also healers who understood that there is a Divine power that infuses the great cosmic energy dance and represents the highest life principle in all of us. Their techniques consist partially in the use of magnets and partially in the use of the natural electrical potentials and polarity in one's own hands, as described in their book: *The Rainbow in Your Hands*

The story began back in 1936 through one of those cosmic and karmic 'accidents' that are an integral part of our destiny and set the seeds for an entire lifetime. Davis

---

[1] Davis died some while ago, while Rawls is still living.

had his own private laboratory even in those days when he was just out of high school and awaiting entry to the University of Florida. He had already been experimenting with little success, to see whether electromagnetic energies affected living organisms. On this occasion, however, he was preparing for a fishing trip and unintentionally left two boxes of earthworms at either end of a large horseshoe magnet, with a third at some distance away. Work in the laboratory became absorbing, however, with the fishing trip getting postponed, while the earthworms remained in their waxed cardboard boxes for the remainder of that day and night. The following morning, however, Davis noticed that the worms had eaten their way out of the container placed against the south pole of the horseshoe magnet, while the other two boxes were undisturbed.

This event set him thinking and experimenting. After innumerable trials that later involved rodents and other animals, he was able to conclude that both the north and south poles of the magnet had distinct, but different effects.

After a twelve day experiment, Davis recorded that the south pole earthworms were extremely active and were approximately one third larger. The presence of young worms in the soil showed that baby worms had been born.

The north pole earthworms, on the other hand, had fared badly – many had died and those remaining were thin and showed little activity.

Davis was using magnet strengths of between 100 to 4500 gauss in his experiments, moving quite rapidly to the use of long bar magnets because of their polar separation. The earth's magnetic field is about one half a gauss, so the field strengths used represented a considerable energy input over the natural background to which living organisms are attuned, and this factor should be born in mind when appraising their results.

Davis analyzed various biochemical aspects of his results, noting, for example, that the ability of the south pole earthworms to metabolize amino acids into proteins was enhanced, while the metabolism of north pole earthworms was depressed. Control experiments were, of course, always conducted to establish the norm.

Davis moved on to testing the effects of exposure on

seeds treated before planting to north or south pole energies. The seeds responded in a manner similar to the
earthworms – the south pole plants germinated more
rapidly and were bigger and stronger than the controls,
while the north pole plants were smaller.

Biochemical analysis of the plants whose seeds had been
exposed to south pole energy for only a short period of
time showed an increase in carbon dioxide intake and
oxygen output. Absorption of nutrients was increased and
root growth was enhanced. 'Sugar beets yielded more
sugars. Peanuts presented outstanding increases in oils,'
writes Davis.

Davis' experiments, later conducted with the help of
Rawls, have spanned over forty years. They have checked
and double checked their results. They have presented
theories and practical results of experiments conducted on
the nature of magnetism – their work on the nature of
electron spin and the north and south pole energies has
already been briefly discussed.

Their findings on the different effects of the two magnetic fields can be summarized as follows:

The north pole slows down and relaxes the processes of
life. Thus, application of a north pole can be used to
control pain by depressing the sensitivity of the nerve
endings. It will also lower the blood pressure and correct
the growth of cancer cells. Their experiments with rodents
showed an extension of life related to a retardation of
maturation and growth, added to which was observed:
'An upgrading of all their sensitivities, including intelligence, reflexes and environmental reaction, inferring the
brain's ability to be more sensitive in recalling information
and responding to their environment.' (*Magnetism and its
Effects on the Living System*). The north pole when applied
to the forehead is also reported to increase ESP sensitivity,
as well as calm down the rational thinking mind, though
we do caution against this as a means of mental control and
development. There are other safer ways to proceed than
the use of high or even low energy magnets.

The south pole, on the other hand is a strengthener and
promoter of growth. Rodents reared after exposure to a
south pole, prior to the early stages of development,
showed increased life-span, vigour and vitality. They also

tended to be oversexed and required to be kept away from others. In particular, the depletion of strength in the male, reacted on the heart and other organs resulting in a decreased life span. South pole rodents, however, were duller and slower witted.

Amongst humans, when applied to the forehead, the south pole stimulates the mind, leaving it in a less calm state.

These differences of effect have led to investigations of the most appropriate orientation in which to sleep and it is not surprising that clear, refreshing and relaxing sleep is best achieved when one's head is pointing to the north and one's feet to the south.

Davis and Rawls' experiments did not end with magnetism. They were quite naturally interested in the electrical polarities present in the body and these they were able to map. Two of their charts are presented here, but they do point out that although the basic relationship of positive to negative is fixed in normal, healthy subjects, the individual voltages can and do vary. The charts represent averages.

Note immediately the similarities of polarity between these findings and those of Dr. Stone. The left is negative with respect to the right, the front is positive with respect to the back. Note, too, the points of zero potential or electrical balance or change-over, in the body.

Davis and Rawls found that the negative electrical energies of the body were related in nature to north pole magnetic energies, while the south pole energy had correspondences with positive electrical energy. This is immediately apparent from a brief study of the alkaline and acid balance in the body. The balance of alkaline and acid in the body is of paramount importance. An imbalance will lead to dysfunction and disease. Alkaline conditions contain the OH^- combination in greater abundance than the acid, ie. H^+ ion. O is oxygen and H is hydrogen and note that the balance or neutral point of electrical ion activity is in the combination of the two: H^+OH^- or H_2O, our old friend water – the universal solvent of life's processes – the balancing or neutral pole, the satvas guna.

Acid conditions create the nervous, hyperactive individual and so does the application of positive electrical

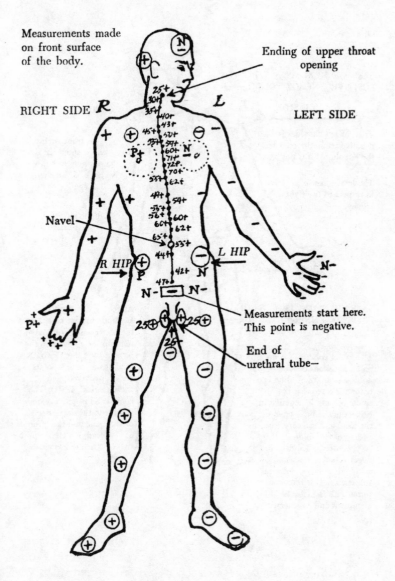

Davis & Rawls chart of bodily electrical potentials – Front surface

137

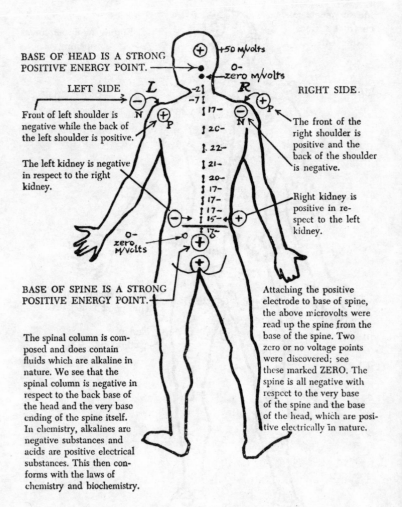

BASE OF HEAD IS A STRONG
POSITIVE ENERGY POINT.

+50 m/volts

0-
zero m/volts

LEFT SIDE *L*

R RIGHT SIDE.

Front of left shoulder is
negative while the back of
the left shoulder is positive.

The left kidney is negative
in respect to the right
kidney.

-2
-7
17-
20-
22-
21-
20-
17-
17-
17-
15-
17-

The front of the
right shoulder is
positive and the
back of the shoulder
is negative.

Right kidney is
positive in re-
spect to the left
kidney.

0-
zero
M/volts

BASE OF SPINE IS A STRONG
POSITIVE ENERGY POINT.

The spinal column is com-
posed and does contain
fluids which are alkaline in
nature. We see that the
spinal column is negative in
respect to the back base of
the head and the very base
ending of the spine itself.
In chemistry, alkalines are
negative substances and
acids are positive electrical
substances. This then con-
forms with the laws of
chemistry and biochemistry.

Attaching the positive
electrode to base of spine,
the above microvolts were
read up the spine from the
base of the spine. Two
zero or no voltage points
were discovered; see
these marked ZERO. The
spine is all negative with
respect to the very base
of the spine and the base
of the head, which are positive electrically in nature.

Davis & Rawls chart of bodily electrical potentials – Back surface energy or the south pole of a magnet. But the overly-acid person burns himself out and ends up with high blood pressure, stomach ulcers and similar ailments. Acidity also relates to clockwise, centrifugal, expanding electron spin and the rajas guna of activity.

Alkaline conditions correlate with negative, soothing, electrical and north pole magnetic energy. The electron spin is anticlockwise, centripetal and cohering, leading to stagnation. This is the activity of the tamas guna of inertia. Note, too, the calming and positive effect of negative electricity in the shape of negative air ionization.

There is yet a further fascinating piece of the jigsaw puzzle provided by Davis and Rawls. Tomatoes, normally an acid vegetable, had their level of acidity reduced when the seeds were treated with north pole magnetic energy prior to germination, making them more palatable and less irritable as a food to those of an already overly acid constitution.

How does this energy get transmitted through the seed to the growth and qualities of the plant? How is the exposure of rodents and earthworms affected by an exposure to magnetic polarity long after the exposure has ceased? The answer perhaps lies in the electron and particle spin and the motion created at this early stage of development in the primal energy patterns that constitute the vibrational energy blueprint out of which the organism develops and has its being, in the basic energy vibration in its more subtle state. Remember, the cases of illness due to exposure to radiation that do not manifest until fifteen or twenty years later, that we mentioned in the previous chapter?

Davis and Rawls, together with Dr. Stone, were among the first to point out that the healing techniques used in the 'Laying on of Hands' and built by Dr. Stone into a powerful therapy, have a direct correspondence to the electrical polarities of the hands and the parts of the body where they are placed. A mother, for example, will place the front of her left hand (negative, soothing) or the back of her right hand (also, negative, soothing), on the forehead of her child (normally negative). This has a soothing and calming effect on the child. Similarly she may instinctively apply her right hand palm (positive) to the upper part of the spinal nerve column or the back of the baby's head (both positive). This also has a calming effect. Man is not the only species to apply these techniques. Primates have been observed to exhibit similar behaviour.

What the mother is doing is using the natural polarities of her own hands to balance the polarities of the baby. She is supplying her own energy to balance that of the child. And this is the basis of all healing with hands, added to which are the effect of the more subtle energies and the quality of vibration in the healer, including their mental attitudes and intentions. Every element, molecule and atom has its own unique vibration and emanations – electromagnetic and more subtle and these vibrations pass between us and influence us in our daily life. This makes it very important, therefore, for any healer to have a well-balanced being and have healthful energy about them, both to influence their patients as well as resist the negative effect that certain of their patients may have on them.

So this is the work of Davis and Rawls. They have provided us with a lifetime of research into the more physical aspects of the effects of magnetism and electrical potentials. This work deserves to be taken up and studied in great detail in relation to the healing arts in order to determine in what ways we may use polarity-based devices, as well as our hands, in order to create healing. Dr. Yao's Pulsors which we discuss next are a step in this direction.

In fact, there are a number of uses being made of magnetism in modern healing therapies, some of which are discussed in chapter 7.

Bio-Crystal Pulsors® and The Work of Dr. George Yao

In order to better understand the significance in the work of Dr. Yao, it is good to know something of the influences and background which have shaped his thinking.

George Yao was born in China to one of the first Catholic Chinese families, in 1922. During the time of the revolution, his family escaped to Hong Kong and became a part of the banking fraternity. George graduated from university as a chemical engineer and after working in Hong Kong for some time on the earliest applications of stretch nylon, he went to work in California as an aerospace engineer for Hughes Aircraft. There he gained much experience and studied further in molecular physics, including special materials and crystals used in electronic engineering. He worked extensively on materials to cover the re-entry modules of the first American satellites.

Later, he left Hughes Aircraft and graduated as a naturopathic doctor, also studying Polarity Therapy and Acupuncture. The combination of his eastern background, plus all these talents and interests, led him ultimately to the development of Pulsors®.

The first Pulsors® were created around 1970 and have been in a continuous state of development and refinement since that day. Dr. Yao told us one day that the Pulsors® were created originally as Christmas gifts for his friends to put on their TV sets. However, they wanted more and insisted on paying, which left him with a small business on his hands. His manufacturing has been increasing exponentially since that time and I can well understand it. His Pulsors® really do work and the world is greatly in need of this kind of antidote to electromagnetic pollution and the general effects of stress and unhealthful living. Perhaps, a hundred years ago, they would have been a luxury, or their effect unappreciated. Now we have a more subtly aware element amongst us and an environmental problem of enormous magnitude.

While realizing the significance of the work of Davis and Rawls on the use of magnets, I have always been concerned about the extremely high gauss that they have been using. This is justifiable for research purposes, but for therapeutic purposes, especially in those without serious illness, the use of such high power is likely to be unnecessarily dangerous. Whenever one applies energy from without to the body's system one is likely to create side-effects. It is far better to work with the body's own energies and create the desired effects by natural amplification. Indeed, Davis and Rawls, themselves express caution concerning the strength of magnets and the duration of exposure utilized. Just for comparative purposes, it is worth noting that the miniature magnets used to stimulate acupuncture points and meridians are about a quarter to a half a gauss in strength, similar to that of the earth's natural magnetic field – while Davis and Rawls were using magnets between 100 and 4500 Gauss. Had they studied the energy meridians and flowpaths, it is likely they could have achieved the same results by the more specific and finely tuned application of magnetic energy of much lower gauss. But how does one set about studying and treating the energy flowpaths of seeds, worms and rodents?

Dr. Yao, however, is working at finer or more inward energy levels, using resonance, rather than the application of outer power to achieve the desired effects. The result is a subtle system of treatment, using devices – Pulsors® – that automatically synchronize with the body's energies, amplifying and cleansing them in a way that no magnet can and enhancing the effects of 'Healing Hands.' When the subtle energies are thus energized, healing automatically begins to take place.

There is no doubt that the interaction of energies between therapist and patient is of considerable significance even with Pulsor treatment, but it is quite normal for the large part of a therapy session with Pulsors® to be passive. The Pulsors are put into position and the therapist, after following certain procedures and hand movements with Pulsors, then leaves the patient with the Pulsors in place, though he may move them into different configurations as time progresses, to achieve specific or general results.

What then are Pulsors®? Dr. Yao explains that a Pulsor consists of millions of microcrystals that have been designed and processed in such a way that they can act as energy resonators – receivers and transmitters of energy at specific frequencies. When placed on the body, or within the body's energy field, these crystals tend to organize themselves into geometric patterns – receiving, amplifying and re-transmitting the body energies with an ordered pulse of their own. Hence the name Pulsors®. The body energies are thus amplified – Dr. Yao suggests up to two or three times, according to dowsing evidence – and energy congestion and disharmony are dissolved. This results in a feeling of great relaxation both physically, emotionally and mentally. They also remove the jangled and tired feeling that some people are aware of after working with electronic equipment, computer terminals and so on.

Dr. Yao also comments that Pulsors seem to be capable of absorbing the multitude of free electrons that are present in our body, especially in those of us in contact with electronic equipment, when watching television or even switching electrical power on and off. Free electrons and free radicals or bits of molecules, especially those carrying a charge, are known to do damage to body biochemistry and are a significant part of the ageing process. This is why people take anti-oxidants, (many of the vitamins, for example, especially vitamin C) which mop up the free radicals. Various toxins, pollutants and ionizing radiation are also responsible for the formation of free electrons and free radicals.

The exact process by which this absorption of free electrons happens in the Pulsor is not clear – one researcher suggests that they simply remove the charge from electrons converting them to neutrinos, which is an interesting possibility. The Pulsors themselves do not, however, become charged, so the energy of charge must be dissipated in some more subtle manner. Certainly, Pulsors remove the disharmonizing effect of working with electrical equipment and they also seem to make machinery operate more smoothly when placed upon points of energy distribution – electrical or otherwise. One assumes that this latter effect is due to energy alignment, perhaps at a sub-atomic level, resulting in less friction and imbalance. Dr. Yao suggests that they align the spin of electrons in a harmonious manner.

These Pulsor micro-crystals – Dr. Yao also calls them 'quasi' or 'semi-intelligent' crystals – are contained in small discs of varying thicknesses and strengths, about one and a half inches in diameter. They are also compressed into pendants with natural stone finishes and there is a pointed pendulum, the Acu-Pulsor packed with the crystals, that can also be used for stimulating the acupuncture points or working on reflex points in the feet and hands.

Based on his background of study with Dr. Stone, in acupuncture, plus general naturopathic, radionic and scientific research and experience, plus an advanced skill as a dowser, Dr. Yao has mapped the polarities and flow patterns in the subtle energy field he calls the Vortex Energy field. Here we find many old friends. There are mental, emotional and subtle physical or etheric energy circuits. The polarities that drive these circuits are related but opposing to the electrical polarities already described. Thus, the right hand front of the body is negative while the left hand front is positive. There is a switch at the spleen and liver centres, an opposition or toning that links the mental circuits to the etheric through the emotional energy operating at this point. The back of the body is the reverse of the front and the chakras have alternating polarities associated with them, also being different between man and woman. Thus the female reproductive, sacral centre is negative and receptive in subtle terms, while the male centre is positive and outgoing. These alternations continue all the way up – a woman has a positive heart, while man is negative, for example; but a woman has a negative throat centre and a man is positive.

It is immediately obvious that these polarities differ from the electrical polarities discussed by Davis and Rawls and the 'electromagnetic light wave' and functional polarities of Dr. Stone. And there are reasons for this. Firstly, the vortex energy polarity centres are a part of the subtle blueprint out of which electrical energies are derived and just as a mirror reflection of yourself has your right and left sides transposed, so too does energy transpose when it reflects or crystallizes outwardly. Secondly, and related to it, positive and negative are in some degree, relative terms. Thus we say that the soul is the positive force with respect to the mind, which is negative; but in the body, the mind is the positive power with respect to the physical energies which are negative. Then, within the physical energies we have positive and negative polarities.

Polarity, remember, is the differential in energy patterns, the essential duality that results in movement, vibration or flow.

Thus, Dr. Yao comments that the Pulsors are a monopole device – they are all positive from a subtle point of view, unless specifically created otherwise. Yet, because of frequency differentials within the Pulsors that relate to mental, emotional and subtle physical vibrations, it is possible to create circuits, in the same way that a +5 volt energy flows to a +3 volt level to create equilibrium. Though both are positive, the +3 volt acts as negative with respect to the +5 volt.

Exactly what Dr. Yao means by monopole, from a scientific point of view, is not made sufficiently clear by him, because a one-sided coin would certainly be unique. From experience I would say that what is meant is that the effect is always harmonizing, always (from a value-judgement point of view) positive. Remember that there is confusion over the use of negative and positive as, for example, yin and yang, or as value judgements. If something is meant to have a negative polarity, then to make it so or maintain it as such would be a positive step.

The subjective experience of Pulsor treatment is almost invariably one of very deep neuro-muscular relaxation in which healing continues to take place long after the Pulsors have been removed. People feel nourished and warmed in all ways. We have also had many instances of their seeing lights within themselves in flowing and beautiful colours. One gentleman experienced a rainbow of colours flowing up his back and out of his shoulders, with a number of other energy flow visions, experienced as colour. He can, in fact, see part of the flow of subtle energy in his body. He is able to describe in similar terms the flow of energy being created by his acupuncturist.

Because they rely for their effect upon nature's already existing energies, Pulsors can also be used in the environment to amplify positive energy and correct negative atmospheres. They are also used to correct energy disturbances due to electromagnetic radiation. We have them around our house, on the electricity and telephone input, as well as carrying them on our persons. People also put them on water main inputs and around their offices. Therapists use them, not only to enhance the effect of their own treatments, but to protect themselves against the negative energy that they pick up from their patients. Many therapists, especially those doing body work, feel drained at the end of the day because of negative energy transfer. Pulsors help prevent this from happening by amplifying and toning the energies of the therapist so that negativity has no place to lodge. The result is that the therapist feels better, is more open and understanding to the patient and is thus more successful.

We have friends who have them round their swimming pool. Water has an affinity for subtle energy and acts as a capacitor or storage medium, and the atmosphere in the pool house has thus been considerably enhanced. Water as pools or streams in a garden gives a peaceful vibration to the environment. It is the balancer of acid and alkaline, positive and negative, and spreads its subtle influence, though water running beneath a house drains the dwelling of positive energy and can cause health problems and a bad atmosphere in the house. Similarly, areas of negative earth energies are associated with ill-health and unhappiness amongst those dwelling there. Pulsors have been used with considerable success in all of these applications in harmonizing discordant vibrations and negative energies.

There are, of course, many people using crystals and minerals in a variety of ways to induce healing. However, much of their work relies heavily on the individual's own natural healing power and energy. This is true of all healing work, whether it be herbalism, homoeopathy or crystals, though the extent of its relevance varies from therapy to therapy. Pulsors represent the simplest and most powerful way of using crystals that I have yet encountered. A simple science and methodology has been worked out that allows one to get started. From there, one's own intuition and experience become invaluable guides.

From a subtle energy point of view, the monopole aspect of Pulsors makes them unique amongst crystal-based devices. This ability to determine the subtle energy polarity is part of Dr. Yao's breakthrough. If you take an accurate pendulum like the Acu-Pulsor over a natural mineral crystal, you will normally find multitudinous changes of polarity over its surface, while the surface of a Pulsor is all positive. Pulsors differ, too, from normal mineral crystals in that they cannot be 'programmed' to a particular vibration, in the same manner in which many crystals are used by healers. They will channel, harmonize and amplify subtle energy, but they are their own boss! It would probably be quite difficult to psychometrize a Pulsor that had been cleaned of any exterior fingermarks, etc. Psychometry is the ability to determine the past history of an object from its subtle vibrations.

Indeed, a psychically-gifted friend of mine, on holding a Pulsor for the first time experienced a feeling of great warmth and energy emanating from it. On the suggestion that psychometry would be impossible with a Pulsor, she commented that it was her habit to psychometrize articles she held, but with the Pulsor, she could not tell anything of its history. Just that it was warm.

Summary

Dr. Randolph Stone, Davis and Rawls, Dr. George Yao – three pioneering approaches to the use and understanding of the essential duality in nature to promote healing. Because it requires a philosophical or cosmic understanding to appreciate the profundity expressed in the simplicity of their findings, their work is often overlooked by many conventional scientists. But as we move into the twenty-first century and science becomes enlivened by an understanding of basic cosmic patterns of energy interchange, so, I believe, will the research of these pioneers be seen as epoch making in its influence.

Pulsor® is a registered trade mark of Yao International.

CHAPTER 6

Crystals, Resonance and Modern Physics

In the chapter on Polarity and Harmony, we touched on the relationship of subtle energies to sub-atomic structure and movement. In this chapter, we expand the theme and show how crystalline matter has a unique arrangement of sub-atomic energy and could be expected to influence, regiment and harmonize matter in both the sub-atomic and pre-sub-atomic or subtle states.

Sub-Atomic Structure

Starting from without and moving inwards, we observe matter in three dimensional form, structure, density, colour and sound. Its density makes it solid, liquid or gaseous and the movement of its atoms and molecules also gives rise to the sensation of heat or cold. Its interaction with the area of the electromagnetic spectrum we know of as light gives it colour, perceived through the eyes. Its ability to resonate and vibrate gives rise to airborne wave forms, interpreted by our ears as sound. We also take cognisance of certain molecular relationships and structures through our organs of taste and smell. Some moths are so sensitive in this respect that they are aware of only one molecule of a pheromone (sex-chemical) emitted by a female, over thirty miles away. Of all the states, conditions and relationships in matter, our senses filter out only a tiny fraction of the available data, presenting it to us as our 'objective reality'.

Taking a step inwards, we find that matter is composed of molecules, some large – some small. Each molecule is composed of atoms. Each atom, until the advent of modern physics, was considered to consist of a nucleus of positively charged protons and zero-charged neutrons, with a number of 'shells' of orbiting electrons.

Thus our solid matter is mostly space in which the particles are moving so fast that, like the whirring blade of a propeller, they appear solid. In fact, if a propeller was flat and rotated fast enough, it would appear to be as solid and flat as a disc of metal. If it oscillated rather than rotated, it would also have all the characteristics of being stationary. You could even bounce a ball off it. It is an interesting fact that super-high speeds of oscillation or vibration have the appearance and properties of being still.

In fact, modern physics does not stop with the classical theory of atomic structure. When we probe deeper we find that the macroscopic parallels and observations of our sensory perceptions do not hold up in describing the structure of sub-atomic matter. Our basic, building blocks of atoms become less solid the further we investigate. They are considered as wave packets, as electromagnetic force fields, as energy relationships. These particles have properties, not all of which have parallels in the macroscopic world of our senses. They have 'spin' – they rotate about the axis of their movement. They have an 'oscillation', like an ultra-high-speed pendulum. Whilst spinning and oscillating, they move around relative to each other, in three dimensions. They also have an 'electrical charge' and a 'magnetic moment' and therefore an 'electromagnetic field'. They have qualities known to physicists as 'strangeness', 'colour' and 'charm'.

Some of this movement has been quantified. The nucleus of an atom vibrates at about 10^{22} Hz, that is 10, followed by twenty two zeros, times per second. An atom vibrates at about 10^{15} Hz. Molecules oscillate at around 10^9 Hz, while living cells vibrate at around 10^3 Hz.

This means that no two atoms, molecules or sub-atomic particles will be the same, because their movement and properties, which change and vary, are an inherent aspect of their existence. Indeed, the very fact that they are separate spatially, means that they are different, just as two identical items in our macroscopic world are not the same. Each has its own unique existence.

Futhermore, the ultra-high speeds of sub-atomic energy approaching the speed of light require physicists to involve the use of Einsteinian relativity theory as well as Quantum theory in their search for valid mathematical models.

Basically, relativity theory considers the physical universe as a four dimensional 'space-time continuum', where movement (spatial relationships) and time (change of position relative to a specific 'frame of reference') are integrally connected. At low relative speeds of movement, the time aspect can be considered as something fixed and independant of the object in three-dimensional space. This is the basis for classical Newtonian physics.

However, it should be pointed out that all theories in the realm of sub-atomic physics are indeed only *theories*. No existing single theory or mathematical model covers all the known or experienced phenomena. Indeed there are a number of theories vying for a place in accepted scientific circles. Thus, for example, there are theories that see the 'fundamental' particles not as points but as extended objects ('superstrings') or as vortices of whirling energy. Such theories are mathematically more complex, but are appealing from a vibrational point of view, though even the 'conventional' theories also see their particles as being in constant motion, as vibrating.

Resonance.

Leaving this train of thought temporarily, let us introduce another aspect of the matter, that of resonant or harmonious frequencies. If we stretch a wire between two fixed points and pluck it centrally, it will vibrate with a wavelength equal to twice the distance between these two points.

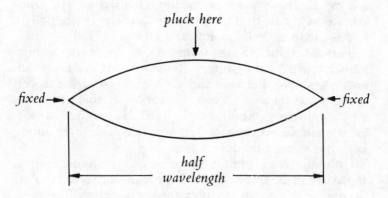

pluck here

fixed →   *← fixed*

*half
wavelength*

If we pluck it at a quarter of the distance along, it will vibrate with a half of the original wavelength.

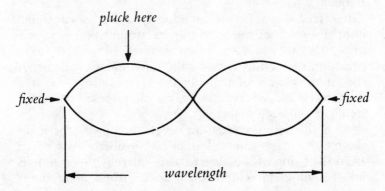

Similarly with other points along its length that provide equal divisions of the string.

These waves create analogous patterns in the molecules of our air, which we call sound waves and which are capable of interpretation by our ears. Hence they are known to us as sound.

The basic wavelength of the string is called its resonant wavelength, the other potential waves are other octaves or harmonics. All musicians who have studied the science behind their art will be well aware of these relationships. Generally speaking, harmonious music is that composed of wavelengths of the same or similar families. Discordant or disharmonious music comes when notes or wavelengths of sound from different families are played together.

Note that our metal wire is vibrating in effectively one dimension. If we now take a metal plate, clamp it at one edge and draw a violin bow across one of the free edges, it will, like the string, emit a note. If we place some light, dry sand on the plate, we will notice that the sand moves to take up specific patterns on the plate. What is happening is this: the plate is vibrating (this is what causes the sound) in two dimensions and the sand is moving to the places of minimum or no movement, analogous to the nodes in the one-dimensional vibrating string.

Note at this point, that the length of the wire (and also its density, diameter and tightness), or the dimensions of the plate, dictate the nature of the wave produced. In other words, each wire or plate will have its own natural frequency.

In fact, if you, quite randomly, knock with your knuckles some of the solid objects around you, you will notice that they all emit different notes, but that the note or sound each emits remains the same unless you change the circumstances of that object – for example, what is touching it and where, etc. This is the resonant or natural frequency of each object.

At high relative speeds, however, the kinetic energy of the moving parts can no longer be considered as separate from the being of the object itself. There is, for example, no such thing as *still* light. Light or electromagnetic energy moves, inherently: it is part of its being what it is. Similarly, there is no such thing as a *still* electron. Part of its being is movement.

Everything – large, small, molecular or sub-atomic has a natural resonance – an easy and natural way of being. And everything – large, small, molecular or sub-atomic can be made to vibrate at dissonant or unnatural frequencies as well as at frequencies that are harmonious with the 'basic natural resonant frequency'.

To summarize our thinking thus far:

1. All matter is energy patterns of sub-atomic relationships and interconnections, moving at tremendous speeds, the speed being an integral aspect of matter itself.

2. All objects have both natural harmonious vibratory frequencies, and can also be made to vibrate at dissonant frequencies, disharmoniously.

As we discussed in chapter four, it is the nature of the movement of energy at the sub-atomic level which gives rise to the harmonious or disharmonious, to the positive or the negative aspects of health and environment. Indeed the word 'disease' means just that. It is 'dis-ease', lack of ease or harmony.

We suggested that the positive or negative polarity in the subtle fields is related to the direction of rotation of sub-atomic particles, clockwise or anti-clockwise, and pointed out that without the cessation of motion – which would mean the ceasing to exist of the particle in our physical world – the direction of movement (and hence the polarity) of the particle can be changed.

However, it is the balance of clockwise and anti-clockwise, of positive and negative that makes up a harmonious or disharmonious energy pattern. For harmony, both must exist in a balanced state. And since no particle can exist on its own, but only in a complex cosmic web of energy inter-relatedness, including other polarity aspects, (eg. its electrical charge), the harmony or disharmony must be considered within an entire lattice of sub-atomic energy. This means that the harmony or balance at one point will have a direct bearing on that at another. That is, *harmony or disharmony can spread.*

This is exactly what we observe in our macroscopic world. If we hum a note of the same frequency as our stretched string would emit when plucked, it will begin to resonate – picking up its movement from that of the sound waves in the air molecules surrounding it. If we hang a number of pendulums of the same length on a wall and start them off oscillating out of phase – that is at different points of their to-and-fro movement – after a time they will pick up on the minute vibrations in the wall and perhaps the air, and all move into phase-resonance. This is the easiest, most natural and most harmonious state for them to be in.

If we now starting hitting the wall with a hammer, creating waves of frequencies dissonant with our pendulums, their behaviour will become dissonant and out of phase.

This tendency towards harmony and disharmony, we can observe in many aspects of our life. It is said that a number of women living together in peace will begin to menstruate at the same time. We have all noticed how the powerful presence of one loving and harmonious person will bring harmony to a group, often without their saying or doing anything. Similarly, some people are essentially disharmonious in the atmosphere they create around them.

It is therefore valid to theorize that the harmonious or disharmonious state of movement among the sub-atomic energy patterns is a part of the process in the creation of the duality and pairs of opposites observed in our macroscopic world.

There is another odd natural phenomenon exemplified by the expression: 'It never rains but it pours' that deserves discussion here. While I was writing this chapter, a friend dropped in, commenting that way beyound the bounds of co-incidence, both their electric toasters had gone wrong simultaneously. These clusters or wave-like patterns in co-incidence of like objects and events are a real natural phenomenon. Lyall Watson in his book *Supernature*, describes how the biologist Kammerer, 'Spent days just sitting in public places noting down the number of people passing, the way they dressed, what they carried, and so on. When he analyzed these records, he found that there were typical clusters, things that occurred together and then disappeared altogether.' 'This kind of wave pattern', Watson points out, 'is familiar to all stockbrokers and gamblers, and every insurance company runs its entire business of assessment on similar tables of probabilities.'

Kammerer was only one of many people who have made it part of their life's work to collect information on coincidences of this nature. He was so struck by it that he called it The Law of Seriality.

It all fits together with our discussion of rhythms, resonance, harmony and duality. Like attracts like – they are easier together, more in harmony. Like also can create like by inducing sympathetic resonance. Like will also repel dislike. Some cosmic rhythms we accept naturally: the movement of the planets, day and night, temperature and weather, artistic and musical harmonics. Life is not all 'equal' – certain things belong together, others do not. People of similar kinds seek each other's company. Everything has rhythm and movement. It is all a part of the law of karma – cause and effect in the cosmic energy dance.

Crystalline Matter

The unique aspect of crystals is that they are solid matter in which all the atoms and molecules are ordered and structured. This is what makes a crystal different from any other lump of solid matter. For example, a pure crystal of table salt, sodium chloride, $NaCl$, is a perfect cube. This reflects, exactly, the basic arrangement of the atoms of sodium and chlorine that make up the molecule of sodium chloride. They are arranged at the four corners of a cube, thus:

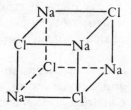

When a crystal is being grown in a solution of table salt, the molecules fit themselves together in the most harmonious way possible and ultimately become visible as a solid cube.

Similarly, other molecules have different basic shapes and this is reflected in the shape of the crystal that can be grown from them.

This harmonious and ordered structure of energy patterns in a crystal is used by modern science in a number of ways, the most well-known of which is the piezo–electric effect. To understand this effect, we must refer back to our discussion of electrons moving in 'shells' or 'orbits' around the nucleus. Electrons can be in outer or inner orbits. The energy of an electron is higher when in an inner orbit than in an outer orbit. If we force the electrons into an inner orbit and then allow them to jump back into an outer orbit, the difference in energy is given off as electromagnetic radiation, part of which is visible as light. The energy can also be given off as an electrical potential.

Modern electronics, by applying an electrical potential to specially prepared crystals can produce a highly accurate, fixed frequency, pulsed electrical potential from crystals, this being the basis of crystal radio frequency generators, quartz wrist watches and so on.

Another way of making a crystal emit light is by physically compressing it, pushing the electrons into an inner orbit, and then releasing the pressure. As the electrons move orbit, energy is emitted as electromagnetic radiation, part of which is at the visible wavelengths of light.

The modern range of cigarette lighters make use of

crystal compression to release energy making an electrical spark jump across the gas outlet, causing ignition. These are the flint-less lighters, a very thin sliver of crystal being used.

This discussion of the piezo-electric effect is to give some idea of the uniqueness of crystals, which is based on the highly ordered structure of their sub-atomic and molecular matter.

For example, a crystal of corundum, pure aluminium oxide (aluminium and oxygen atoms arranged in an ordered fashion) is colourless. However, if some of the aluminium atoms are replaced by chromium atoms, the crystal takes on a red colour and we call it a ruby. The chromium also introduces an instability or acts as a negative catalyst to the growth of the crystal, thus explaining why almost all rubies are always of small dimensions. In fact, two of the worlds largest and most famous rubies, the Black Prince's Ruby and the Timur, both in the British Crown Jewels, are not rubies at all, but red varieties of spinel. Similarly, a true blue sapphire is again corundum with traces of titanium. When other elements are also present in the crystalline structure, saphires can be purple, pink, yellow or green.

Now, returning to our observations of resonance, we can easily understand how the natural harmony and order present in crystals can create resonance in neighbouring sub-atomic energy vibrations, causing the effects with which we have become familiar in our use of Pulsors. Pulsors, in fact, are an ordered arrangement of billions of microcrystals laid down in a very specific manufacturing process, designed to create harmony and resonance wherever they are placed.

Pulsors are, perhaps, like a sergeant-major. If you place a sergeant-major amongst a homogeneous, disorganized assortment of raw recruits, it will not take long for this one highly organized and strong centre of energy to induce order into the previous rabble! He will make them resonate with his own natural pattern of being.

We can now understand, therefore, how electromagnetic radiations can affect us for better or worse, at the sub-atomic level, because matter is no more than energy patterns, taking on the appearance of solidity. Its sub-atomic structure is of essentially the same nature as electro-magnetic radiations. It is held together in atoms and molecules by forces which are akin to electromagnetic radiation. We can therefore expect matter to be affected by all aspects of electromagnetic radiation (and also gravity and magnetism). It may not change its outward shape or appearance, but its inner motion is almost certainly af-fected.

Indeed, we already know that high frequency cosmic rays can disturb the atomic structure so much that new elements are created. Should we not expect radiation at other frequencies to be changing the inherent vibrational energies within matter? Elements differ, sub-atomically, only in the number of electrons, protons and neutrons they carry in their atoms. Hydrogen, for example, has the smallest and lightest atom, comprised of one proton 'or-bited' by one electron. Helium is a little heavier, with an additional neutron. This also makes it a more stable atom, less inclined to combine with other atoms in the manner of hydrogen, which can sometimes do so explosively. Other elements simply have more electrons, protons and neu-trons in their composition.

And here are two more every day phenomena that have to be understood at a sub-atomic level. Firstly, objects have different colours... How? The energy that makes up the object, when 'hit' by electromagnetic radiation at the frequencies of light, absorbs some wavelengths and re-flects others. Why? Think about that! It is a truly dynamic, sub-atomic world in which we live!

Secondly, the ordered structure of energy within many crystals, allows electromagnetic radiations at the wave-lengths of light to be *transmitted*. Crystals are transparent! The more perfect the crystalline structure, the more per-fect its transparency. Flaws create disturbances in the transmission of light, light is selectively reflected and transmitted by surfaces and changes in density. If you grind the crystal up and try to look through it, it is opaque. Light is not transmitted. And then, of course, crystals absorb some wavelengths and transmit others giving them the appearance of colour, these colours of crystals also being caused by impurities in their structure. It is all very fascinating.

It is said that the Atlanteans used crystals as their sources of power. We are now beginning to understand how this could be. The energy within matter is enormous. Einstein's formula is that the energy available is equal to the mass times the square of the speed of transmission of electromagnetic radiation, $e = mc^2$. Crystals can already be made to emit light and electricity, but to do so, an external source of energy has to be applied. Pulsors are used to harmonize energy, but no exterior light or kinetic energy is emitted.

If we could create an unstable crystalline structure that spontaneously emitted electromagnetic radiations at the frequency of light, while moving into a state of stability, we would have a remarkable device. The essential component of a solid state light emitter! Another approach might be to 'charge' a crystal in some way, the charge being slowly released as visible light.

If this sub-atomic, kinetic energy could be released as kinetic energy, we would then have a crystal powered motor! So-called nuclear power stations and nuclear explosions are nothing more than a massive and highly dangerous way of transforming 'solid' matter into other forms of energy (heat, electricity, etc.) The side effects are devastating and the long term effects on our health, even of 'safe' nuclear power stations is indeterminate.

We, as a human race, are so bound up in the world economics of energy that changes are difficult and the more subtle effects on our well-being are easily overridden by the short-term economic interests of the governments and international businesses involved. It is significant that safety standards are normally increased due to pressure from environmentalists and rarely from within governments and industries themselves. Money, power and self-esteem make humans very short-sighted! The essential human situation of ignorance gives us a tendency to obscure this reality by trying to feel that we know a lot! The fact is that despite all scientific description, we still do not know what makes the sun come up in the morning! For this understanding, perhaps a mystic, inner kind of knowledge is required.

Gem Remedies and Colour Healing

One can also understand that it is in a similar manner that gem remedies and colour healing work. The inner vibration of the crystal has certain qualities, as does light or colour of a particular wavelength. These vibrations will have healing qualities wherever that vibration of energy is required as nourishment by an individual. The vibration can be transmitted readily to pure distilled water, being the point of balance, chemically and electrically speaking, and thus we have a remedy as a pure vibration. Similarly with colour healing where the vibration is applied through the use of filtered light energy. This, too, is how homoeopathic remedies have their effectiveness. Analyzed chemically, scientists proclaim that their is nothing there – and especially with the remedies prepared radionically, through the use of vibration pure and simple. It is the quality of subtle movement and vibration that constitutes the remedy, not the chemical aspect. So unless the laboratory can analyze that movement, its analytical procedures are incorrect for the substance supplied and its 'findings' are hence invalid. Lack of understanding of the correct approach does not constitute a reason for criticism or condemnation. Galileo, Keplar and many others could testify to that!

The application of specific energies to key parts of the body such as the foot or hand reflex points or acupuncture meridians by means of crystals, Pulsors, mini-magnets, needles, pressure electro-acupuncture, colour or whatever, will also, clearly, magnify the input effect of the vibrations.

Hence we can understand why doctors recommend wearing certain rings on certain fingers for specific problems or general toning of particular body systems. In some Eastern traditional medicine, the gems are even ground up and taken with the food, so that their vibrational influence may permeate throughout the bodily, emotional and mental energies. We have also heard of rubies and other precious stones being ground up in order to tint the glass used in the creation of colour healing sanctuaries.

Sub-Atomic Fingerprint

Let us end this chapter with a further hypothesis, not proven, but one that makes a lot of sense and is definitely possible. It is the experience of many of us that some people are good with mechanical objects. Machines, cars, electronic equipment all work well for them – we touched on this in a previous chapter. Other people are a disaster area, equipment is always breaking down around them!

We also know that there are energy pathways between physical objects, including our bodies, and our emotions and thoughts.

Could it not be that the vibrational movement patterns of sub-atomic matter are automatically affected by our thoughts, moods and being? A harmonious person will induce harmony into the sub-atomic energy dance, while a disharmonious person will automatically create disharmony.

This is reflected in the overall performance of the equipment and explains how a harmonious person like George Yao could drive his sports car for 100,000 miles without a service, especially since both his natural resonance and his car were also re-inforced and amplified with his Pulsors!

I have also noticed how an angry and disturbed person will have equipment go wrong around them, whereas when calmness is present, the equipment works more smoothly. Sometimes, the careful and loving dismantling and re-assembly of a faulty piece of equipment will be enough to make it work once again, without one ever knowing what was wrong!

Furthermore, this hypothesis explains a number of other phenomena as well. Psychokinesis is the ability to move physical objects around through the energy of thought alone. This, of course, requires a movement of sub-atomic energy patterns in order to create a total movement of larger objects. Some experimenters, therefore, wondering whether it would be easier for their subjects to move sub-atomic particles, set up such an experiment using radioactive emissions, with a Geiger

Muller counter as the measuring device. The result was that subjects with psychokinetic abilities were able to make higher scores when moving beams of sub-atomic particles than in moving larger objects.

Since, in our mystic understanding of the cosmos, we perceive a vertical continuum of energy which at its lower end links the energy of thought and emotion with the subtle and gross physical energy patterns, through the movement of energy at the sub-atomic level, the result of the above experiment is quite understandable. It simply requires less effort or mental energy to move sub-atomic particles.

It is both a predictable corollary and an observed fact, that subjects working in laboratory trials of telepathy and psychokinesis, report – sometimes extreme – mental depletion after experiments. They have simply lost mental and probably emotional energy.

There is a further aspect of this hypothesis. People who are sensitive to atmospheres are also frequently aware of the vibrations of objects. Objects in a person's environment and indeed the whole environment itself take on a vibration that is akin to the person or people living there. This is experienced by many people as 'atmosphere'. Part of this feeling is no doubt in the subtle energy content of such vibrations. However, since all energies are interconnected, could not the physical manifestation of these subtle energies be found in the sub-atomic energy movement patterns?

This would explain the psychic ability of certain people to know some of the history of an object simply by holding it in their hands and inwardly tuning in to its 'vibrations'. Psychic people have called this ability 'psychometry'.

In other words, we are all leaving a unique fingerprint in the sub-atomic energy patterns as we go through life. It reflects back on us in a variety of directly mechanical and more subtle, mood-affecting ways. We are all living in a psychic and mystic ocean, but with only the barest tips of our noses into the clear air of consciousness and understanding of what is going on!

Crystal-Based Technology

Many crystal researchers have reported allied phenomena. Telepathic ability is enhanced when certain crystals are held in the hands or placed on the persons involved. Crystals can be programmed to contain a thought-induced image or even mood, thus allowing psychometry by other individuals. Some experimenters even 'programme' a crystal to be a meditative mood inducer, using it to help in their meditation. Some have shown how telekinesis is enhanced when crystals are used in the experiment.

In the *Crystal Book* by Dale Walker, many interesting thoughts are put forward. To quote:

'We can charge a crystal with energy and the crystal will store that energy for later use. Our experience has shown we can store information in a crystal. We do not have an adequate test to prove this. Remember in the Superman movie the crystal with all the knowledge which taught the baby and later the man? We are working on the techniques for recording and recovering thought-forms stored in crystals. As an example, consider the crystal skulls found in Central America and believed to be such storage computers by many crystal researchers. These researchers have seen visions of all ages and found that they have become aware of new knowledge after working with the crystal skulls.

Regarding the use of crystals in Atlantean and Lemurian science, he continues:

'Our research channeling spoke of a whole civilization of incredible power and splendor made possible by crystal science. Machines were merged with the power of the mind. Crystals were used to furnish unlimited free power. They were used to convert the sun's energy into a form of electricity. We saw pictures of alternating concave and convex lenses catching and changing the rays of the sun and storing the changed energy in a liquid material. We later identified this as a solution of liquid crystal.

'Great grids were designed to capture and use the energy field of the earth. All were powered and made possible with crystals.

'Through the use of controlled thought to direct the chemical changes of matter, huge crystals were grown in very exact shapes. Even the molecular design was changed to shape and direct energy in exact ways. Sound and light were mapped out in precise frequencies not only physical, but mental as well. These were fed through these designed crystals to power air, sea and undersea craft. The discovery of the use of crystals to control the incredible energy reaction between matter and anti-matter gave birth to space flight. When they linked this drive to the ability of the crystal to assist the mind to travel interdimensionally, they were able to design interstellar space craft and fly to the stars.

'Crystals were used in construction. We saw a picture of a circle of people around a crystal. All of the people had been trained since childhood for perfect concentration. We could see a beam of energy travel miles away to a workman holding a box with a lever, a control stick on top. He pointed it at a huge stone, moved the lever and the stone rose and poised in the air. Another slight adjustment and he walked away, moving the stone in front of him.

'Large towers like lighthouses were erected near the sea. Operators were stationed here to communicate with the dolphins, porpoises and whales. With their assistance, the operators herded large schools of fish into waiting offshore nets.

'Mighty and beautiful healing temples filled the land. Here the combination of light, colour, sound, magnetism and thought energies were channeled through crystals to create wonders in healing.

'The Atlanteans mastered the intricacies of all the rays and sub-rays of color and sound. They mapped the neurological pathways of the human body and brain. They knew all the energy channels of the energy bodies. Etheric surgery on the energy body was preferable and more desirable than on the physical. When it was necessary, priest healers linked with the minds of the patients to direct the cells of the body to separate and expose an offending organ. Blood vessels were directed to close off. Cells around the organ released their hold and forced the organ to the surface of the body where the healer took it out and placed it in a rejuvenation chamber. When the organ was rebuilt, it was replaced in the body. The cells reconnected themselves, the blood vessels sent blood back into the organ and the wound closed itself up. There was no pain, no bleeding, no infection and no shock.

'Some perverted the great good the crystals were designed to do. The power of the crystals was used to destroy and enslave. The tremendous energies released caused an inbalance in the earth. A massive earthquake brought about the total destruction of Atlantis.

'Some survivors took the crystals to other lands. In Egypt, they built a towering pyramid, using crystals to lift and set the massive blocks.

'They used the laser-like energy to cut and dress the blocks so precisely a folded piece of paper could not be passed between pieces of stone weighing tons. They made the base from granite, knowing the weight of the stones above would squeeze the quartz in the granite to generate an energy field which they used for healing, rejuvenation, and religious ceremonies. They sheathed it in sandstone and chalcedony to form a resonator and capped it with pure quartz. With this gigantic transmitter, they were able to keep limited communication open with their friends in the Pleiades and the other star systems.

'Wherever the survivors went they left records. They left them beneath the Great Pyramid in Egypt, in caverns in the Tibetan mountains, and in pyramids in China, South America and North America. Mountain peaks all over the world also have their depositories. They left tablets of a man-made stone, hard as diamond. They left books of gold and thousands of crystals.

'The real information was in the crystals where 200,000 years of knowledge of one of the mightiest civilizations on earth was stored as 3-dimensional thought holograms. These crystals will be found and deciphered before the end of this century.'

Unless one has direct experience of something, there is always an element of doubt about its validity or the motives or reliability, however sincere, of those describing their experiences. Deception, too, and glamour, are an intrinsic part of astral vision, but the fact is that we are here where we are. There is so much for us to learn – and so much prejudice and pre-conditioning to unlearn. Each one of us is on a personal odyssey, so let us open our hearts to understanding wherever we can. We are all very human, we just need to follow our star wherever it leads.

With regard to the use of higher forces to control physical matter, for myself, I do not believe that one should waste mental or even spiritual energy in the conscious attempt to perform what are, essentially, miracles. All such energy is precious to us. Should it not be used only for inward, spiritual and mystical advancement? Spontaneous telepathy and so on, are a natural outcome of spiritual awakening and should become a natural part of one's being, without much energy being consciously directed to develop it. Ultimately, our own life and being are our only real possession, and it is our inner spiritual and mystic awakening that should be of paramount concern to us. This is the fuel energising mind and matter.

CHAPTER 7

Subtle Energy Interface, The Bioelectronic – Biomagnetic Body

No mention of subtle energies is complete without discussion of the aura. All the subtle energies of living creatures can essentially be considered as a part of their aura, though in the strictest sense, it is considered as the energy emanating from or surrounding them. Indeed, even after the life force has departed, materials made from natural living plants have a vibration more pleasing and harmonious than artificial substances. Compare, for example, the feeling of wood, cotton and wool with nylon, polyester, vinyl and other plastic materials.

Our consciousness or soul is encapsulated in a sea of energy interconnections which we observe through our five physical senses. The entire universe is simply a dance of vibrating energy. And all physically perceivable matter has its finer, more subtle counterpart. In life forms, because of their inner connection with the Great Source, these subtle energies are an integral part of their expression in the energy fields of creation.

These energies are appreciated by sense organs of the same vibratory nature as the energy being experienced. Thus our five gross physical senses perceive gross physical matter. And just as subtle energies are the blueprint for less subtle energies, so too are our senses a part of a vertical spectrum of senses that perceive the motion and differences of energies along this spectrum. Thus, when reading descriptions of auras, they are seen, apparently with the eyes, though sometimes even when the physical eyes are shut. Similarly, in psychic, astral and mystic experience, sight, sound, feeling, aroma and taste are all involved, but in their more subtle states.

In fact, being aware of the aura is nothing more than an awareness of energy at whatever level or vibratory rate, that aspect of the aura is being experienced, through the awakened senses at that level. This, of course, gives us an understanding of why the aura is variously and sometimes conflictingly described by different people. It depends upon what energy field or vibration, the attention of the observer is fixed and it may also depend upon the individual too, as to how he describes his experience. And in the realm of the subtle, *the influence of the observer* upon the experience is more immediate than at the grosser level.

So the observer interacts with what he observes: to one degree or another, the subtle connections and interplay will always be there. His personality and karma will always influence his perception. Thus, a person who is truly happy, inwardly, will make other people happy just by his presence, while the miserable person will spread his misery wherever he goes, probably complaining as to why everybody else is so miserable! In human relationships this modification of each other happens continuously and is part of the adjustment we all make in any relationship, consciously or unconsciously.

It is also true that the stronger personality will also influence the weaker. The one will be made to resonate with the other. Strength of character and especially spiritual strength is always reflected in the aura, in its size, quality and harmony. Many folk have experienced the atmosphere of people and places, though frequently the energy aspects of this phenomena are not appreciated. Sitting next to a peaceful and loving person will uplift one, while being near an upset, disharmonious or angry person will pull you down. Similarly, a bright, warm, sunny day in spring, when the flowers seem to blossom with a scintillation of colour and their fragrance fills the air, uplifts your heart with the energy of new life bursting forth in nature. There is subtle energy almost visible. If you half close your eyes and tune in, you can almost see the vibrancy of new life, surging all around.

In the animal kingdom, this awareness of vibration seems almost second nature. It is a sixth sense, an instinct we say, that warns them of danger or moves them towards food and pasture. No doubt, some creatures may have other gross senses, perceptions of change in the gross physical environment, that we do not possess, but subtle aspects seem to be strongly present too, to anyone of an observant eye.

Amongst the so-called primitive cultures, all but obliterated now from our planet, telepathy and an inherent ability to tune in to the vibrations of each other and of nature and its forces were very much a part of their way of life. The Australian aboriginees spoke of 'leaning on the wind', the African bushman – read *The Lost World of the Kalahari* by Laurens van der Post – communicated telepathically with each other at a distance. The Kuhunas of Hawaii and certain 'priests' from other cultures in the South Pacific have a naturally developed psychic awareness and capability.

In the more sophisticated cultures of the past, the Chinese, the Indians and the Tibetans all developed forms of Yoga and meditation, specific internal exercises to open up mystic or perhaps just a more psychic consciousness. The Tibetans, especially, are famous for their 'seven-league-psychic-boots' – moving at high speed over land by manipulation of natural forces. Some of their cliff-ledge monasteries can only have been built by use of natural forces yet to be harnessed and understood by modern physics. There are authenticated reports of modern witnesses to ceremonies in which large blocks of stone were moved through the air up onto cliff ledges, for building purposes. Indeed, there are many stone circles, a vestige of ancient European cultures, where the stones are known to have come from far away, by a means yet unknown. If one brings in a knowledge of subtle energies, then many new possibilities and explanations emerge. One hesitates to mention the Egyptian pyramids, in this respect, the subject of every possible theory under the sun, and claimed by almost every occult philosophy – which only goes to show just how unclear their purpose was, as well as their method of construction.

After all, moving a large heavy object or even one's own body is only difficult due to the force of gravity. And what is gravity? An inherent attraction of matter to matter, of energy to energy, one of the basic forces of nature. But what is its essential and innate nature? What *is* it? Nobody can give an answer in scientific terminology that allows one to design some method of controlling this force . . . yet.

Similarly with modern research into telepathy, for example. There are many, many people in our modern age, who have an understanding and awareness of vibration and atmosphere. They may not be totally telepathic or clairvoyant, but they are definitely partially so. It is a bi-product of meditation and other practices that stimulate subtle energy awareness and control – Hatha Yoga, Ta'i Ch'i, Pulsors, Reiki to name just a few. Such folk are mostly quite uninterested in helping research scientists to prove or disprove the existence of these subtle energies. It would be like men with eyes in a blind community, helping the blind research whether or not sight actually exists! It is useless knowledge to the blind people, even supposing they could believe the possibility of sight – which most of them would not. They would just offend the sensibilities of the sighted ones. No doubt, the magicians amongst them would soon show that they could, by subterfuge, do the same things as the sighted ones, which doesn't prove very much at all, except that a few blind people can pretend to have sight and fool some of their neighbours. It would be far better for the sighted ones to keep quiet and keep company with the others who have sight.

And this is indeed what happens. Human beings who have developed themselves this far are naturally reluctant to spend hours of their precious life in a laboratory trying to guess numbers or cards. In fact, the scientists involved in this kind of work are often themselves, consciously or unconsciously, seekers of a higher reality. Their work and research being simply an outward expression of their inward need. This includes even the antagonistic ones – perhaps especially them. Love and hate are, after all, but two sides of the same coin. A fish, once hooked, may come to land with ease or it may fight. But either way, there is no escape for it.

Molecular and Heat Auras

And so we have a spectrum of energies – physical, emotional, mental and higher – all with a presence within the human aura, and all capable of being perceived and often of being confused with each other. At the gross, physical level, there is a molecular 'aura' extending from the body a few inches, composed of keratin (skin) particles, tiny salt crystals, ammonia and other organic materials and gases. Then, there is electromagnetic energy, in the form of infra-red radiation – heat. Modern thermographic analysis equipment can detect disease in the inner organs by an analysis of the infra-red patterns emitted. Within this heat envelope are also a host of bacteria and micro-organisms which probably breed there too. Warm air currents are drawn up towards the mouth and nose and its contents re-introduced into the body. Apart from the more obvious advantages, this fact underlines the importance of regular bathing and general cleanliness in the maintenance of health.

The Body Electric

There is also an electric field around the body extending at least a few inches. This field of pure electrical potential was first discovered by Professor Harold Saxton Burr at Yale in the 1930's and described in his book: *Blueprint For Immortality*. This field, which is set up around all living creatures at an early stage of their development, probably from the point of conception, reflects changes within their physical and psychological make-up that are manifest now or which are likely to happen in the future – a tendency towards such a condition.

Professor Burr demonstrated relationships within this field to the electromagnetic variations in the sun – sunspots – as recorded over many years on trees within his University campus.

He also discovered that there are changes in electrical potential at the time of ovulation during a woman's fertility cycle, as well as noting differences in the electrical potential of seeds that were destined, genetically, to become vigorous or stunted in their growth. Professor Burr conducted many such experiments over a period of many years, indicating that these potentials accurately reflect, conditions within both the body and mind, including cancer. He concluded that these patterns of electrical potential were *primary* and in the nature of a *controlling* field. That is: changes in this field *determine* changes within the body – that the field is not a secondary effect of bodily changes, but that it comes first. Furthermore, he found that these potentials responded to external environmental electromagnetic stimuli – magnetic storms, sunspots, solar and lunar variations and so on.

It might be relevant to point out here that sunspots are no small event. They are nuclear events, little understood, about 200,000 kilometres in diameter, about fifteen times that of the earth, and emitting a barrage of particles and electromagnetic oscillations that reach us on earth within only a few minutes. They are directly responsible for radio interference and electromagnetic events in the earth's atmosphere – thunderstorms and the like. Indeed the background level of emission of solar particles, the solar wind, plays an integral part in the weather and atmospheric conditions on earth, also being responsible for the Northern Lights or Aurora Borealis. Sunspot activity is also correlated to times of disturbance in the earth's history, in an eleven year cycle. These events being both social – wars, times of unrest, etc. – as well as geological and meteorological.

Burr's work has, in recent years, been followed up by a number of American scientists, Dr. Robert Becker in particular, nominated in 1978 for a Nobel prize for his pioneering work on the effects of electricity and electromagnetic radiation on living organisms. The story has many threads and the total picture is not at all clear, but the narrative includes both Burr's work and also that of the Hungarian-American biologist Szent-Gyorgyi, who was awarded a Nobel prize back in 1937 for his research into metabolism. Szent-Gyorgyi suggested that cellular and other living tissues might have semi-conductor properties in the manner of electrical and electronic components. This idea of electronic activity within living creatures is supported by many strands of evidence, including research into the homing mechanisms of pigeons. Pigeons, it seems, have a number of navigational systems. Not only do they have a prodigious line and distance of sight covering many miles, but they also use the sun, stars and the earth's geomagnetic field as alternative navigational systems. This means that they are sensitive to minute magnetic changes and disturbances. Furthermore experiments with pigeons in artificial tunnels with only magnetic cues to enable them to find their way to food, revealed that they could do so, but only if they were able to flap and flutter their wings. The answer to the functioning of this geomagnetic navigational mechanism seems to be that a bird's feathers contain the protein keratin, which is thought to have piezo-electric properties, the movement of the pigeon's wings being necessary for the generation of an electrical impulse directly related to the nature of the magnetic fields, thus allowing them to appreciate field strengths and direction.

Keratin is also found in hair, animal horns, hooves, skin and nails as well as whiskers – those highy sensitive organs possessed by cats and many other creatures. Compare them, for example, with the antennae of moths and other insects. The piezo-electric effect is also known to exist in bone and other tissue, not due to the ionic mineral content, but due to electronic phenomena within certain protein molecules and probably the cellular structure itself. And DNA itself, the genetic chromosomal material, is also known to have piezo-electrical properties.

It would seem highly likely, therefore that man's nervous system is far more than an enlarged domestic wiring system, but is a super-bioelectronic, biomagnetic system of electromagnetic fields and forces, currents and charges with information gathering, storage and retrieval functions, a million times more advanced than any of our modern computing systems. Robert Becker's work, for example, has included partial regeneration of limbs in rats – bone, muscle and all the other tissues – simply by the correct application of electrical pulses, potentials and polarities.

In fact, Dorothy Hall once told us the story of a young lady who suffered from epileptic siezures. This girl had long, long hair – a mane, her boyfriend called it. Dorothy Hall tried everything and also sent her to every kind of practitioner she thought might be able to help, but to no avail. Finally, the clue came in a chance moment when the patient commented that only once, after she had had her hair cut short, had she had any relief from epilepsy. Well, her boyfriend was wild when her hair was cut, but it cured the epilepsy. I would also have been interested to know whether the epilepsy was worse when in the vicinity of electrical appliances or whether any such cabling ran behind her bedhead.

Along similar lines, one of our daughters has had her hair 'frizzed' a couple of times and on both occasions they have been followed by a period of emotional imbalance. And if you have ever seen hair under the magnification of an electron microscope that has been permed or even treated with certain cosmetic hair preparations, you will see a sight from a horror movie. The hair looks like weeds after they have been treated with hormone weed killer – tangled and contorted in structure, quite unable to perform any energy exchange or balancing function that might once have been expected of it.

So if hair has more to its function, as we are suggesting, than thermal control and cosmetic value, then one can understand how its electrical properties, when connected to the scalp and acting as a medium for the input of energy to the brain, can modulate brain function or, when connected to the body can act as one of the mediums for general energy exchange with the environment, both for nourishment and information gathering.

There are, indeed, many phenomena reported by researchers indicating both subtle and gross responses of living creatures to electrical and magnetic stimuli, often of very low intensity. A. S. Presman in his book *Electromagnetic Fields and Life*, suggests that these responses are due to changes in the *information handling* aspects of our bodily electronic system, since the stimuli are too small to make any obvious change to the physiology and biochemistry of the tissues. This accords perfectly with the research of Burr, Becker and others when they postulate that there is a basic controlling aspect to the subtle 'electronic body'. If the controlling blueprint is modified, then regeneration or degeneration of tissues can result, depending upon the change effected.

Thus, there are a number of magnetic and electromagnetic therapy devices available on the market which do help a considerable number of patients. Negative air ionizers are very well-known and have been used not only for clearing up stuffiness due to central heating or closed windows, but also in burn and wound clinics where the flesh heals faster. Most people who have them in their office, living room or bedroom feel a benefit to their mental clarity, as is borne out by efficiency studies conducted in negatively ionized offices, while those with asthma, bronchitis, hay-fever and other bronchial problems often get relief. Emotional stability is affected by the level of positive or negative atmospheric ionization and negative air ionizers can often alleviate symptoms of depression, as well as migraine headaches.

One of the earliest biologists proposing a theory incorporating the vibrational or oscillating aspects of cellular materials, was George Lakhovsky, whose book *The Secret of Life* was first published in English translation in 1939. His thesis was that the nucleus of each cell had the essential characteristics necessary to maintain an oscillating electrical circuit.

Szent-Gyorgyi too, back in the 1950's, noted that the molecular structure of many parts of living cells, might behave as semi-conductors, somewhat in the nature of crystals. Semi-conduction is a phenomenon occurring in materials with a highly ordered molecular and atomic matrix allowing electrons to move from one molecule to another, normally when a certain threshold voltage is reached, giving the electrons enough energy to jump. Szent-Gyorgyi felt that proteins would have this ability and, as we have described, work on keratin as well as collagen (found in many body tissues) has shown him to be correct. Moreover, electron microscopy studies over the last two decades have shown that cells do indeed possess highly complex and ordered structures. Szent-Gyorgyi's idea that proteins may be linked throughout the body into long chains allowing information, coded electronically, to flow along them, has therefore been given some experimental support.

This concept of information encoded into oscillating electromagnetic waves first came into being with the advent of radio transmissions. Lakhorsky, Szent-Gyorgyi and others were simply applying principles recently discovered by physicists, to the human body. Nowadays, with the advent of computer and information technology, utilizing the crystalline, as well as semiconductive and chemical electronic properties of substances such as quartz, silicon, gallium arsenide and others, we can find it easier to imagine that the body has similar information storage and processing capabilities. In fact, it is well known to many biologists that phenomena 'discovered' by physicists and chemists are later found to be already in use in nature either universally or in particular species. Just consider the bat and its radar, the pigeon and its built-in compass, the torpedo fish and its use of electricity and many others besides. Similarly in our concept of the human body. We often 'discover' things in the body when we 'discover' a more outward parallel. In fact, there is no outward human artifact which does not have a biological parallel within our own bodies. The basic mechanisms of energy pattern re-arrangement are all found within living cells and organisms. Consciously or unconsciously, our human artifacts only mimic specific aspects of nature.

Take, therefore, a leap in imagination into the great host of unknowns that go into the processes of life. No scientific 'discovery' does more than provide a more detailed description of events according to certain theories or concepts. This kind of knowledge has only scratched the surface of the potential detail available for observation. Science, even allowing for its in-built restrictions as a means of understanding the greater questions, has only touched the surface of its possibilities. And yet the surprise, inertia, prejudice and even antagonism that greet a new 'discovery' is a feature of human advancement throughout all the ages. History tells us of our errors, but we do the same old thing in a new disguise, not realizing just what we are doing!

So let us re-view and re-visualize our concepts of what our body is and what we are, in our essence. The reality is that nobody knows (except a mystic) how we even bend a finger. What amazingly intricate mechanisms and energies of thought and body are involved in such an apparently simple operation!

Lakhorsky, with his Multi-Wave Oscillator, as well as the more modern Dr. Becker, along with researchers using magnetism, have all reported their ability to influence metabolic processes, as well as mood, for good or ill. Lakhorsky's oscillating electrical circuits were able to enhance plant growth, as well as rid his geraniums of injected cancers. Burr was able to monitor physiological and anatomical changes by measuring his L-field (Life field) potentials. Becker has been able to stimulate tissue regeneration in amputated limbs and induce bones to knit that were otherwise proving problematic. Researchers in

Sweden are treating cancer with small electrical currents. The application of magnetic foils or small magnets to sports injuries, as well as arthritic and rheumatic joints have given much relief to these sufferers and helped the healing process. Electro-acupuncture, the use of acoustic resonances (Cymatic Therapy), Pulsors, air ionizers, magnets and many more such devices and methods along these lines, point inescapably in one direction, whether we find it understandable or not.

It is clear, of course, that there is a positive and negative aspect to everything. Electricity and electromagnetic radiation can also have powerful negative effects as we described in a previous chapter.

Knowing, then, that electrical phenomena are very closely related to effects in subtle energy, we can thus see both a pattern and a mechanism emerging. The complex bioelectronic, biomagnetic body energy pattern is a precipitation or step-down from the more inward subtle energies. This becomes very clear from our work with the Pulsors as balancers of subtle energy disturbed by electromagnetic and other dis-harmonizers. It is also very clear from some of the new acupuncture equipment now available. Acupuncture, as we said previously, is a harmonizing of subtle energies the Chinese know of as Ch'i. The subtle energy fields being dealt with by acupuncture flow along meridians or channels with specific points along their length at which treatment is applied, by means of a needle or heat by burning the herb, *moksha*. The points and meridians relate, reflexly, to the inner organs, systems and general energy balance of the body.

It is known that these acu-points are distinguishable from the surrounding areas by virtue of a drop in the electrical resistance of the skin from as much as one million ohms to as little as two thousand. There are a number of electro-acupuncture devices that detect these points and stimulate them electrically rather than by needle or heat or, in the case of Shiatsu (acupressure), by finger massage. There is also a system of applying small magnets to the acu-points, discussed later in this chapter, from which practitioners claim great success. Dr. Hiroshi Motoyama of Japan has taken this process a step further by designing a computer-based, electronic acu-point analysis system. By attaching an electrode to the terminus of each of the twenty eight meridians, the current flow along each meridian is measured and very minutely analyzed. The computer then prints out an analysis of the body's electrical energy system, indicating the points at which treatment is to be applied, to restore the natural balance.

This measuring of the skin's electrical response as a reflection of the state of the Ch'i was also used by Dr. Pat Flanagan in his pyramid energy researches, where he showed very clearly that pyramids have a balancing effect on these subtle energies.

Electromagnetic Life Energies

It is well established that the nervous system uses electrical activity and emits electromagnetic radiation, mostly at the lower frequencies and especially associated with brain waves and heart function. This is what constitutes electro-encephalograms and electrocardiograms. Modern research, however, has shown that this radiation, far from being a bi-product of electrical nervous activity, may have a fundamental role as an information-laden, organizational energy field.

Dr. Morell, a medical doctor from Otfingen, West Germany, after some considerable research into biophysics, developed his concepts of molecular vibration as a pattern blueprint of bodily function and together with a brilliant electronics engineer, Edwin Rasche, produced the first Mora therapy units in 1975, refinements to which are still in progress. The word Mora is derived from the first two letters of the designers' names.

These two scientists have discovered a wide spectrum of electromagnetic emissions that, they say, relate directly to the molecular vibrations of the individual. This pattern is read into sophisticated electronic analysis equipment from the acu-points, detected by the change in skin resistance. It is then 'cleaned up' – disharmonies removed etc. – and fed back to the patient. The results are quite remarkable and successful.

Associated with the Mora equipment, is a colour therapy unit. Colour has been used for healing from time immemorial, often associated with the colours of the chakras. Even modern psychologists are aware of the mental and emotional relationships to colour – certain colours being used to induce different moods and so on. In the Mora equipment an interesting deviant of this technique is used which relates directly to the electromagnetic aspect of colour. A pure white source of light is generated, within the unit, this light is then split into its three primary components of red, green and blue, by the mixing of which, the secondary colours of green, violet and orange are produced.

The colour chosen for the patient is then converted electronically into a lower electromagnetic frequency bearing a harmonic relationship to the original colour. This is then used for treatment purposes.

Similar in certain respects to the Mora equipment is the Indumed magnetic field device, developed by Dr. Ludwig of Tubingen, also in West Germany, after research dating back to 1963. The first clinical models were available from 1974 onwards, following research at the University of Freiburg. 'Indumed' is derived from the words Induction Medicine.

As we have pointed out in several places, we live in an environment in which natural electrical and magnetic phenomena have a considerable role to play. Between the ionosphere and the earth's surface, there is a voltage gradient of about 200,000 volts of static electricity representing a differential of about 400 volts between your head and your feet when standing outside in the open air. This electrostatic field is not constant, but varies, containing within it vertical oscillating waves of a fundamental, basic frequency, modulated with many harmonics, the whole having a sequence repeating several times per second. These harmonics extend into the megahertz range and have a regulating and stabilizing influence on physiological processes.

These Schuman waves, as they are called, are a natural part of our environment that are blocked or reduced by many modern building materials and urban environments. Furthermore, for Schuman wave formation, a reasonable level of conductivity is required on the earth's surface. This conductivity relates to the ground water level which in recent times has been reduced through use in industrial applications. Thus, cities, for example, are places of low or absent Schuman wave activity.

In healthy people, the absence of Schuman waves can be tolerated, but in sick people, there is greater need of their stabilizing effect. The absence of Schuman waves is also felt by those under stress and Schuman wave generators are one of the devices used by NASA to keep their astronauts in good psychological condition.

Also permeating our natural environment is the lithosphere – the earth's magnetic field modulated by electron-plasma waves and ultra-fine energies emitted by trace elements. The Indumed equipment employs magnetic field generators that use iron filament impregnated with these trace elements. The result, along with other refinements to further mimic the natural electron-plasma and Schuman waves, is an instrument that has considerable power as a therapeutic aid across the whole range of human health problems. The research shows that different bodily conditions have different rates or harmonic frequencies, and thus the Indumed instrument has different settings for various conditions. All of this correlates very well, of course, with the findings of radionics which identifies specific vibrational rates with particular organs, diseases and conditions. Some psychics, too, are well aware that different organs, physiological and anatomical, systems and conditions have specific colours as perceived by their subtle sight.

Treatment time using Indumed is about fifteen to thirty minutes per session, but if the Indumed output is fed into the patient after combination with output from the Mora therapy instrument, then not only is the treatment enhanced, but it then takes only three or four minutes to produce the same effect. *In other words, the closer we get to harmonizing the individual's natural energy vibrations within, then the less energy we need to create a deeper and more pronounced effect.*

This is something conventional medicine, for all its good as well as ill, should consider deeply. It is the same in all aspects of life. A big result is not directly equatable to the amount of energy and resources expended. What is required is the right amount of energy, at the right time and at the right place. If you push a swing at the right moment, it will go higher with a minimum of effort, at the wrong moment you can stop it dead or break a wrist. Similarly, wealth is not achieved by the number of hours spent in work, but by the correct application of energy. In healing, to create the maximum effect, go to the highest energy level that you can without having to use your own mental or spiritual energy to make the harmonizing adjustment. Or, in more light hearted vein, if you want to be a lazy healer, work with subtle energies.

A personalized version of the Indumed therapy equipment is available as a $2'' \times 2'' \times \frac{1}{2}''$ disc, known as Mecos. Mecos is an electrostatic field generator that mimics the earth's natural electrostatic field with switch selectable modulations between 3 and 30Hz – more or less the range of basic brain wave frequencies. Both myself and a number of friends have personally experimented with this device and found the 3Hz operation to be highly relaxing and soporific, while the 30Hz frequency is greatly stimulating. Although our tests were by no means a thorough scientific scrutiny, we did of course perform double blind tests on each other, to overcome the obvious psycholgical aspects. Case histories from West Germany have shown Mecos to be of use in allieviating pain, including rheumatism, arthritis and migraine headaches and, curiously enough, phantom limb discomfort.

The phantom limb symptom – apparent sensations by an individual in a limb that has been amputated – is of interest. There are, of course, neurological explanations for the effect, but in addition to this, psychic people report that after a limb has been amputated, some of the subtle energy aspects of the limb remain in place. That is, the subtle energy blueprint is still there. This gives hope to researchers into limb regeneration, for if the pattern is still intact, all that is required is to coax the tissues to grow back into the jelly mould.

Returning to our study of bodily emanations, cell division also produces low intensities of ultraviolet radiation which may be a carrier of information, encoded into its modulated wave pattern. The Mora therapists would certainly agree, pointing out that it is not only the ultraviolet radiation which can contain vibrational patterns relating to health or disease, but a far wider spectrum of electromagnetic emissions. The research that brought the possibility of ultraviolet cell communication into prominence was conducted by a Russian group from Novosibirsk, headed by Dr. V.P. Kaznachayev. Some researchers have claimed that cellular ultraviolet light emission induces division in neighbouring cells. Kaznachayev and his colleagues took this a step further. They set up two identical tissue cultures in separate, sealed, transparent containers with a quartz screen in between, the significance of the quartz being that it transmits ultraviolet light, whereas regular glass does not. They then contaminated one of the cultures with a lethal virus and noticed that the *other* culture also showed similar signs of disease. However, when they put a screen of *regular* glass between the two cultures, the uncontaminated culture got along just fine. The conclusion was that the modulation or information encoded into the variable vibration of the electromagnetic ultraviolet emission was able to disrupt the functioning of the cells in the uncontaminated culture.

Hill and Playfair in their book: *The Cycles of Heaven* where some of this research previously unpublished in the English language, is described, go on to point out that that if this encoding is a general part of living organisms, it would be possible to broadcast the electromagnetic equivalent code for a disease, in order to induce its symptoms at a distance. A horrifying thought! Though similarly one could broadcast patterns that relate to health, happiness and well-being. One is once again reminded of the Russian woodpecker signal described in a previous chapter, and wonders just what is its purpose.

This bioelectronic, biomagnetic energy system that we are suggesting – a highly elaborate information storage as well as communications system, with energy links both to the gross physical as well as to more subtle energies – can also readily explain how colours (electromagnetic radiation) can affect us both physically, emotionally and mentally. The use of colour in healing is an ancient art used in both ancient Eastern cultures as well as in modern day therapy. It also explains how full spectrum, natural lighting, makes people feel and work better, as well as helping their immunity to disease, facts well established by the users, researchers and manufacturers of full spectrum lighting.

A theory put forward by John Evans of Cambridge in his book: *Mind, Body and Electromagnetism*, soon to be published, is another expression of the bioelectronic, bio-magnetic blueprint or subtle energy interface. This *morphogenetic* or *morphogenic field* as he and other theorists have called it, is backed up by some interesting theoretical research. Evans has postulated the existence of certain fundamental electromagnetic frequencies along the spinal column and then using modern computer graphics mapping techniques has plotted the contours that relate to the equipotentials or points of equal voltage that would surround the body given these frequencies. The results are quite fascinating, the most immediately obvious aspect being that the contour plots relate quite clearly to both the anatomical structure of the human body as well as the major spinal chakras as focus points of subtle energy distribution (see example).

Evans also points out that while some aspects of bio-logical biochemistry are understood, there is no scientifically expressed theory that explains how living processes are *organized* and relate to each other in a cogent fashion. Clearly a theory that sees the body only as a mass of causually related, billiard-ball-type effects is deficient. Without some master-plan, no such system could avoid resultant chaos. This indeed is true of the world in general, although the pattern behind the apparant chaos may seem harder to determine. It is part of the law of karma. That energy systems require organization from a higher level within themselves is an inherent aspect of creation.

At the biological level, the next higher vibration is in the area of the biochemical–physiological electromagnetic. No greater requirement for this organizational field exists than in the development of embryos into fully formed adult species. Quoting Evans:

'However, for a causal embryological science to develop, we need to formulate an energy field that has the right sort of overall form, is sufficiently complex and variable at the detailed cellular level, and, of course, has some correspondence with experimental evidence. Such a field could only be achieved by an oscillatory organisation of many different frequencies moving continually in and out of phase with each other. Even a single initiating frequency

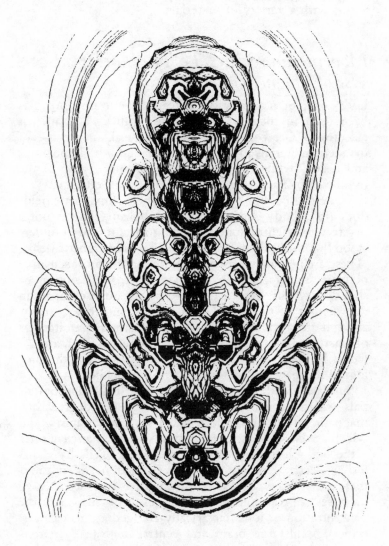

Contour plot of hypothetical equipotentials (according to Evans)

can achieve quite complex patterning, as Chladni demonstrated with sand sprinkled on a vibrating plate. In recent
years, using electromagnetic and sonic vibrations, Hans
Jenny has generated beautifully detailed 3-dimensional
forms with a variety of materials.'

Modern Approaches To The Therapeutic Use of Magnetic Fields

Lodestone, or naturally occuring magnetic iron ore, has
been used in therapy since earliest times. The ancient
cultures of Greece and Egypt both speak of the use of
magnetic materials in healing, including both Hippocrates
and Galen, while the great physician and mystic of the
middle ages, Paracelsus also writes of their efficacy.

There is no doubt that the application of magnetic fields
does affect body energies and metabolism. This is not a
mystery to scientific understanding since it is well understood that the body has its own very weak magnetic fields.
These are normally observable only on the most sensitive
of gauss meters, but in the case of strong emotion or
shock, they can even be detected by a regular compass in
the vicinity of the solar plexus. Cells, molecules, atoms
and sub-atomic particles, in fact all physical manifestations
of energy, have electromagnetic properties that are affected by the presence of a magnetic field. It is the biological mechanisms that are not comprehended.

Similarly, with the effect of electrical fields and potentials which have been studied to a greater degree than
magnetic effects by modern scientists and therapists, and
which are closely allied energetically to magnetic energies
– the one affects and 'creates' the other. Cells have differing electrical potentials or levels within and without
that 'drive' body molecules from place to place. Nerve
impulses are considered to be the result of changes in the
concentration of ions (electrically charged atoms or molecules), whilst the brain and central nervous system is
entirely electrochemical in nature. Indeed, atoms and molecules themselves are vibrating energy fields of electrical,
magnetic, gravitational and other forces. In fact, at a gross
physical level, the body can be seen as a vibrating dance of

electrochemical and magnetic energies, organized by the pranas or subtle life energies into a coherent, operating whole. Without the life energies within, which take their vibrational existence from the mind or antashkarans and which are themselves organized by the soul or consciousness through the heirarchy of intermediate energies, the physical manifestation of our body ceases to exist. When life departs, the complex, integrated organization of body molecules immediately begins a process of disintegration.

The application of energy, force or material substance is therefore, by its very kinship with the body, likely to affect its functioning. Indeed, there is no such thing as *passive* relationships of energy. All meetings are *interactive*. Even one solid object placed upon another is not passive. It is the *interaction* of their vibrating energies that results in the one retaining its shape and sitting on the other. Indeed, if the one is highly energetic it may visibly react with the other. Its weight (force of gravitational attraction) may dent or make a hole in the other. There may be a combining of energies describable at an atomic and molecular level as a chemical interaction. There could also be magnetic or radioactive interaction. The possibilities are endless and if they just *appear* to be passive then this can be understood at a molecular or atomic level by realising that their molecules do not readily mix. A man may have a solid sugar lump on his table for half a lifetime (assuming the flies don't get it), but the first person to put it in water sees its solid structure of molecules interact with those of water and disappear into solution before his eyes. Its apparent permanence as a solid object was quite illusory and entirely relative to its circumstances.

So *all* matter – gross, subtle, mental or higher – exists because it is vibrating and energetic and we can therefore readily understand that magnetic fields and polarity will affect the body.

Therapeutic magnets that are available commercially differ considerably in their strength. The earth's magnetic field, generally considered to be due to ferrous materials within the core, has a strength of about half a gauss, whilst that of the body is many times less. It is interesting to note here, that the earth's magnetic polarity is known to reverse from time to time due to internal and natural causes. And such times are, geologically speaking, thought to be related to periods of considerable biological rearrangement amongst the species inhabiting the earth. There are variations, vibrations or oscillations in this field, too, which are of considerable importance and the more finely tuned a magnet and its associated therapeutic techniques, then the less magnetic energy from without is required to perform healing or balancing of body energies. And naturally, the closer one is to the causative level of energy, the less will be the side effects.

Some magnets are supplied with very little, if any, understanding of the differing effects of polarity. They are usually of higher gauss (sometimes up to 500 gauss – 1,000 times the strength of the naturally occuring earth's field to which we are attuned), and result in a stimulation of the body, perhaps equatable with the use of caffeine as a temporary energy boost. People carry them around their neck or have them loose in a pocket. I would recommend their use only as an emergency measure for acute conditions when there are few alternatives remaining.

Somewhat better is a magnetic foil that is impregnated with a mixture of minerals and mineral salts including iron, potassium, magnesium, sodium, lithium and manganese in phosphate, chloride, sulphate and bicarbonate form. Also included in the mix are silica, copper and zinc. This foil has a field strength of only 10 gauss and yet has an effect as pronounced as higher gauss magnets, with – one assumes – less side effects.

The work of the German scientist, Dr. Wolfgang Ludwig and his Canadian colleague Bigu del Balnco have brought into being a more fundamental understanding of the relationship between what are known as electron plasma oscillations (energy vibrations or waves at a subatomic level) in association with the earth's magnetic and electrostatic fields. These almost subtle vibrations are related to atomic structure, that is – to specific chemical elements and minerals. Taking with them some of the energetic characteristics of their originating element or mineral they spread out using magnetic and electrostatic fields as a *carrier* wave. In other words, the effect of an element or mineral can be transmitted *vibrationally* into the body. This is reminiscent of the mechanisms inherent in homoeopathy, as well as flower essences, gem remedies and so on.

These vibrations are naturally present in the earth's magnetic and electrostatic fields but both the vibrations as well as the fields themselves are reduced within many buildings and urban areas by as much as fifty percent due to the screening effect of concrete and modern building materials. In fact, they are likely to be modified into *unnatural* patterns by building materials as well as by electromagnetic radiation from electrical equipment and cabling. This leads to what many therapists feel is an energetically produced disorientation and deprivation of our source of the earth's energetic nourishment and stabilization.

So the coating of minerals onto the surface of a low gauss magnet permits the vibrational quality of the minerals to be transmitted to the body. Since the energy is thus more finely tuned to the body's needs, less energy is required and a more harmonious energy balance is achieved.

The body, however, has specific pathways – meridians and nadis – through which energy flows as a subtle vibration. Based on the eight extra-ordinary acupuncture meridians, Dr. Itoh of Japan, devised a technique using minimagnets, about a quarter of an inch in diameter and less than half a gauss in strength, to balance the body's energy system. The magnets are used wih a full understanding of their polarity effects. The fundmental principles of yin and yang are well understood by Chinese traditional medicine and even modern scientists know that bacterial and viral infections often take root when the acid-alkali balance (pH) changes within the infected cells. Reversing the 'switch' by restoring the balance of yin and yang (which automatically results in the correction of any pH imbalance) through the use of acupuncture needles or moxibustion (application of heat to specific points) is an ancient Chinese art. Dr. Itoh discovered that this same energy balancing can be achieved through the use of his mini-magnets.

Whether the energy pathways involved in this balancing are identical whether magnets, needles or heat are used (or minute electro-stimulation) is open to speculation. Personally, I doubt it. I would imagine that each source of externally applied energy taps into the energy spectrum at a slightly different point with varying 'flavours' in the net harmonizing result obtained. Indeed, acupuncturists familiar with all these techniques, use them variously according to the needs of each individual patient.

The Biochemical Connection

There is an interesting connection between the body's biochemistry and its bioelectronic, biomagnetic energy system. In fact, it shows once again that we are dealing only with one complex, interwoven energy system; not separable functioning organs and systems, but a unique and wonderful whole.

You may remember the mention in a previous chapter of how the device for detecting induction fields around electrical 50hz AC mains cabling, detects the same electric induction field around the body when someone simply holds an insulated, but live, electric cable. And also that this field is passed from person to person if they all hold hands or touch each other. Our experimentation with this device allows us to see that this electrical *conductance* (ability of a substance to transmit electrical energy) and *capacitance* (ability of a substance to store electrical energy) varies from person to person and from day to day with the same person. We need to do more specific tests, but what does seem clear already is that this *dielectric factor varies with both emotion and the state of health*.

Now, Pat Flanagan reports that he once ate an ounce of pure amino acids (we don't advise you to try it) and noticed that his body capacitance changed in three minutes from 100 picofarads to 0.1 microfarads, a ten fold difference. In other words, there is a direct link between body biochemistry and the bioelectronic energy system. Bearing in mind that one of the major energies responsible for the manifestation of matter is electromagnetic in nature at the intra-molecular and sub-atomic levels, we are forced back to our understanding at the vibrational level, to make sense of these findings.

Indeed, molecular and atomic structures are themselves vibrant, moving energy patterns in which electrical, magnetic, gravitational and other forces are intrinsic. It is only our simplifications in chemical and biochemical terminology and description, along with static pictures and models of molecules and atoms as spheres of 'inert matter' fixed in space that make it difficult for us to see them as vibrating energy structures.

Finally, add in to this train of thought, the specific effects of certain hallucinogenic substances such as LSD and mescalin. The effect these drugs have on the user is dependant upon his own personality and inner make-up, as well as upon the mood in which the drug is taken. This makes individual experiences with these drugs almost as different as those who take them. However, there are certain continually reported similarities between experiences. These include a heightening of physical awareness such that one's *appreciation* of information received through the senses is vastly increased. People feel that they have never before *seen* colours or *heard* music. The vibrancy of colour and sound is enhanced to such a degree that the person will watch in genuine ecstatic bliss the beauty of a sunset or dawn, the movement of clouds in the sky, or maybe just the detail in a painting or a leaf. Even favourite pieces of music are said to be heard with new ears. Users feel that the composer or musician has never before been really appreciated or understood. Taste and smell are likewise enhanced, the fragrance of a honeysuckle, for example, sending currents of real inner happiness through their being.

Time is also distorted. Users of these drugs say that just looking at their watch is enough to make them smile and stare with incredulity. Time seems so slow and in a strange way almost unbelievable. Psychic experiences and telepathic connections with fellow 'trippers' are also frequently reported. Furthermore, the vision of electrical and magnetic fields by clairvoyants, has also been described by users of mescalin.

One should also point out, of course, that hallucinogenic 'trips' can go badly wrong. It seems to need only a small bad experience or thought for the mind to become unbalanced and to turn topsy-turvy, the experience literally becoming a hell out of which there is no escape. I have personally known of people who committed suicide or

became permanently emotionally and mentally unbalanced as a result of LSD and hallucinogenic drugs.
They are certainly not substances to be trifled with for the
sake of a quick high.

But the interesting scientific question is, how do the
molecules of LSD accomplish all this? The heightening of
the senses, the feelings of bliss, telepathic and other subtle
energy experiences tell us very clearly that we are working
on the subtle side of our body's energy system. Either
directly or indirectly, these hallucinogenic molecules are
working through the molecular level to the subtle energies
and our experience with the bioelectronic aspects of the
body tell us that this could be the interface of biochemistry
with the subtle.

A Bodily Crystalline System

At meetings in the USA with trance-channel medium,
Kevin Ryerson, readings were given on the subtle aspects
of healing and health. Ryerson's readings pointed out that
the body itself has a full crystalline system – not yet
properly understood by modern medicine – as well as
biomagnetic and bioelectronic aspects. Included in this
crystalline system are cell salts, fatty tissues, lymph fluid,
red and white blood cells, and the pineal gland. These
crystalline structures operate on sympathetic resonance, as
we discussed in chapter six, and the healing energies of
vibrational remedies – homoeopathy, flower essences and
so on – are amplified in this manner by the body's own
crystalline structures. Similarly, with gems, Pulsors and
Mora therapy equipment etc., the body's energies can be
amplified from 'without' through the biophysical auric
field.

Kevin Ryerson's readings also state that the pineal gland
is a crystalline structure that is an integral controlling part
of the interface between the body and the higher subtle
energies. There is, he says, a constant state of resonancy
passing along the spinal column between two critical reflex
points – the medulla oblongata and the coccyx. This
relates of course, to the energy flowing through the chakras. The information received from subtle energies via
the pineal gland is thus encoded into this resonancy and

information then travels to other parts of the body through the acupuncture meridians, the nadis and crystalline structures, the biomagnetic, bioelectronic energy fields and the neurological and circulatory systems etc. The energy of vibrational remedies, gems, Pulsors and the like activates this entire system, thus affecting the whole of one's health and well-being.

Echoes of this energy system are found in the work of John Evans as well as in Mora therapy research. Specific kinetic vibrations, the minute electromagnetic fields of sub-atomic particles, atoms and molecules, resonance effects, piezo–electric proteins, the electrophysical properties of acupuncture meridians and points, structured bodily crystalline materials – all these present a picture of biophysical energies not readily approachable by modern biochemistry or modern physics at the current time, yet presenting a fascinating and potentially powerful approach to understanding health and healing.

Related work on crystalline patterns has been conducted by the herbalist, George Benner. His interest was first aroused by a book on companion planting – the use of sympathetic energy relationships between plants to mutually stimulate their growth by planting them alongside each other.

Using a method proposed by Rudolf Steiner over sixty years ago, one of the authors, Dr Philbrick, determined the relationships between plants by adding sap from each plant to a 5% solution of copper chloride and allowing the mixture to dry into a crystalline pattern. The pattern for each plant was found to be both repeatable and unique – a fingerprint, so to speak, of that plant's energies.

If the sap from two plants were used instead of one, then the pattern was either harmonious or disharmonious and chaotic. According to Philbrick's research, most plants that are good companions exhibit harmonious patterns, while those not in harmony reflect this in the disharmonious pattern of their crystals.

Benner, being also a botanist, continued this research extending it into the field of at first plant identification and then recognition of pathological conditions by using a drop of saliva from the tongue mixed on a microscope slide with the 5% solution of copper chloride. What he discovered was quite remarkable. Firstly, not only did plants have a unique crystal fingerprint, but the saliva of patients with particular pathological conditions also exhibited this same tendency.

The correlations, however, did not stop there. Benner noticed that the crystal patterns of saliva from people with particular conditions reminded him of certain herbal crystal patterns. On further study, he found that very frequently the herb that is used as a specific for these pathological conditions, accurately matched the condition itself in its crystal pattern. Note that we are talking here of a pattern formed from the saliva of a person with a particular pathological condition. We may be looking at the body's reaction to the condition rather than the disease pattern itself.

If one assumes that the crystal pattern reflects the energy vibration within the material added, then perhaps one can conclude that the body is requesting that vibration in order to heal itself. At any rate, the correlation itself must have some vibrational significance, since it is beyond the bounds of co-incidence.

This subject is endlessly fascinating and my point in raising it is to direct attention once again to the vibrational aspects of energy relationships and their role in the body. The effect of these vibrations upon simple copper chloride crystals is also something of considerable interest. The whole subject deserves further research.

Colour, The Iris, Iridology, Energy and Sunshine

Finally, here is another one of those trains of thought that provide a further piece of the jigsaw puzzle. One might think that colour (electromagnetic energy) or a higher harmonic of it, could have no effect on the body's energy system. But just consider that it is a well-known phenomenon that some blind people can learn to 'feel' colours through their fingers and skin, through touch, and can even describe their qualities. Red, for example, is said to be warming and expanding, while blue is cool and contracting – much as we already react to these colours visually. It means that there is an energy aspect to it, that the vibration of certain frequencies of electromagnetic energy is inherently warming or cooling, regardless of our visual appreciation of its colour. (Note, too, the polarity of these colour differences). Hence the rationale behind the use of colour in healing, in psychology and in sociology.

And note, too, that the reflection or refraction of light at a surface is not a passive process, but is due to an *interaction* of the energies at sub-atomic and atomic levels. At least it can be understood or described in this way.

Now, my wife, Farida, has taught and practiced Iridology for many years. Iridology or Iris Diagnosis is the science and art of diagnosing the state and conditions of the organs and systems of the body, both physical and emotional-mental, from markings and structures in the iris of the eye. Exactly how the iris becomes such a complex map is a matter for much speculation, but there is no doubt that it is. It is the body's instrument panel and one of the major focus points of energy.

What Farida and other iridologists have noted, however, is that not only is the body-emotion-mind complex reflected in the iris but that changes to the iris such as accidents or surgery directly affect those areas of the body that are reflected in those parts of the eye that are damaged. It is thus a two-way system.

Dorothy Hall, the Australian naturopath and iridologist described a number of such cases in an advanced iridology seminar in Cambridge during April 1986. A patient, for example, who had had an operation for glaucoma which entailed the removal of a thin segment from the iris between about 12 and 1 o'clock, subsequently suffered personality changes, mental problems, epileptic fits and other sensory difficulties. And that particular part of the eye relates directly to animation and life, equilibrium and dizziness and certain other cerebral functions.

Similarly, a builder came to her with back problems so severe that he feared he would have to give up his occupation. Dorothy Hall noted a pterigium, (a fatty, vascular growth, common amongst white races living in countries with a strong ultra-violet content in the sunlight) encroaching from the sclera (the white of the eye) over those edges of the iris associated with the spinal area of the body. The growth was removed and *without further treatment*, the back problems completely disappeared.

What this means is that the iris is essentially a reflex zone where energy input can reflexly affect other parts of the human system. It also leads one to speculate that the iris itself is a specific organ with a function of obtaining nourishment directly from light and perhaps from other energies of the environment and the sun.

Indeed, modern endocrinology is already aware of a connection between the eye and the pineal gland that has a association with the circadian rhythm, the twenty-four hour cycle of light and darkness to which we are entrained. And the pineal gland, we also know, plays a master controlling role in the bodily crystalline and subtle energy system.

Thus, the biomagnetic and bioelectronic energy system of the body could also receive nourishment directly from the iris of the eye, specifically related and tuned to the individual organs and systems. From our knowledge of the effect of colour on the body, not just specifically through the eyes, we can understand yet another reason why most of us feel better in the sunshine and when we can get in some sunbathing. And this would also explain why patients who have had their eyes bandaged often become weak, muscularly, even though they may have been out of bed and able to take some exercise. Consider, too, conditions such as glandular fever, two of the symptoms of which are an inability to look at strong light and severe debilitation and energy drain. Perhaps there is a whole area of symptomatic body weakness associated with an imbalance to the energy input system of the irises. It's just an idea, but it would be worthwhile researching.

Nourishment and energy fuel is therefore received by us in many ways, not just by eating and drinking. The organs and systems of the body receive their more subtle nourishment through stimulation of the reflex zones in the hands and feet, as we walk and work, especially if we use soft shoes or the climate and social circumstances allow us to go barefoot. And the iris and body energy system take in electromagnetic and more subtle energy from without by both absorption and resonance.

Summary

As we have previously discussed, modern theories in physics include concepts of virtual or ghost energy. Dr. Shuji Inomata of Japan talks of a 'consciousness-energy-matter' triangle and has derived mathematical formulae that permit understanding of how observable energies of our physical world are manifested out of the 'virtual' or 'ethereal' energy field. He also talks of 'virtual electromagnetic waves' within the virtual or subtle state. This thinking is taken considerably further by scalar electromagnetic theory, which is discussed in the last chapter, but both theories provide a framework into which conventional Einsteinian relativity, quantum mechanics and electromagnetic theory fit, though with certain major re-alignments of conceptual understanding.

In both Inomata's theorizing and scalar electromagnetic theory, vacuum is seen as consisting of real energy in a virtual or subtle state. Modern physics has been aware for a long time that in all observable matter, the sub-atomic particles occupy only a very small part of the total space or vacuum. The new theories see these sub-atomic particles, mass, gravity, electrical charge, electric and magnetic fields etc., as the observable outcome of interactions of energies in the virtual or subtle state. They are like interference patterns between virtual energy waves, manifesting outwardly. They are not separate from the virtual state, but are its observable manifestation, like bubbles on an ocean that exist only because of the ocean, though in our normal physical condition all we can see are bubble patterns, with the ocean lost to view.

In the same way, there is a heirarchy or vertical spectrum of virtual energies, all creating the lower out of the higher, the process continuing up to the level of thought energy and beyond. A clear mechanism is thus described by which mind and its outward projection as emotion, plays on the more subtle physical energies of our being, ultimately manifesting as the outwardly observable energies of our physical body.

The primary morphogenetic patterning of the body thus lies in the mind and the karmas that constitute the fabric of our life, manifesting as a lower harmonic in the virtual or subtle energy fields and finally at the electromagnetic, gravitational, sub-atomic, atomic and molecular level of our bodies. Thus, at all these levels, we will be able to perceive a patterning that reflects life's processes and organization. The deeper the level, the more fundamental the organization, but a pattern will always be there, just as we see DNA and genetic patterns, as well as endocrine and biochemical pathways at a molecular level of observation.

And it is this outward-moving patterning in the vibrating subtle energy fields of 'space-becoming-manifest' that we call the subtle energy interface.

CHAPTER 8

Earth Energies, Feng Shui and Pyramid Energy

Following on from our discussion of the electromagnetic aspects of life, we must also consider the effect upon our well-being of the earth's magnetic and electrostatic fields, as well as its more subtle energies, some of which aspects have already been discussed.

The Earth's Magnetic Field – Vitamins, Herbs & Jet Lag

That the earth has a magnetic field is, of course, unquestioned and knowing what we do about the bioelectronic and biomagnetic aspects of living creatures, it is very easy to see that there will be interactions between living creatures and the earth's magnetic field. Since this field is by no means uniform and bearing in mind other phenomenon such as background radio-activity from rocks and soil, one would expect to find areas that either promote or upset one's level of health and well-being. One can readily understand, too, how high-speed travelling across time-zones, and the earth's magnetic field can cause disorientation in addition to that created by the upset to our 24-hour circadian rhythms.

In this respect, one can also comprehend how high doses of vitamins, especially Vitamin C, are reported to give one strength against these disorientation aspects of crossing the earth's magnetic field. Vitamins and hormones are amongst the key biochemical constituents of living tissues. Their molecular construction is of paramount importance in the energy interchanges at the molecular level. However, as we have discovered, there is a vibrational and subtle content within all matter, also called the life force or prana. Perhaps vitamins are stronger carriers of prana than other substances and at different vibratory frequencies or levels. Thus, when we take vitamins, we strengthen our subtle energy system and, when travelling, we are not so liable to the vibrational disorientation which we describe as jet lag.

It is certainly true that vitamins give us more energy and bounce – increase our Ch'i, the acupuncturist might say – both at our more subtle emotional and mental levels as well as physically. This also underlies why *natural, un-processed* vitamins will be more effective than man-made counterparts. Man may be able to make a molecular look-alike, but he cannot fill its vibrational capacity with pranic life energy. This is true of processed natural vitamins, too: some of the life energy will have been lost, just as it is when food is cooked rather than eaten raw. This gives the underlying rationale to the use of fresh fruit and vegetable juices, which are full of nutrient biochemically as well as being 'pranically' loaded.

An interesting corollary to this is provided once again by recent Russian research published by Hill and Playfair. It has been discovered that certain natural herbs can give protection to living organisms from the effect of harmful radiation. Ginseng root has long been known amongst herbalists for its general bodily *strengthening* capabilities, not just in its popularly known effect on sexual appetite. Dr Breckman from the Institute for Biologically Active Substances in Vladivostok, has reported that just a single dose of Siberian ginseng is sufficient to extend the life of laboratory rats exposed to X-rays. That is, it strengthens their energy systems against the vibrational disruption of high energy electromagnetic pollution. This knowledge of the vibrational and pranic content of the food we consume should make us thoroughly assess what we feed to our bodies and its effect on our health and well-being. Perhaps the day is not so far off when junk foods will carry a government health warning!

The Earth's Electrostatic Field

The electrostatic field of the earth is well confirmed and monitored, though there are many aspects which puzzle scientists. This field, a part of advanced meteorological study, extends from the ionosphere – the region of ionized atmosphere beginning about 50 miles up – down to the earth. The earth's surface is negatively charged while the ionosphere has a positive charge, the potential difference between the two, being in the order of 300,000 to 400,000 volts. We do not feel this charge because we are in connection with the earth and are therefore negatively charged with respect to the atmosphere. The atmosphere maintains a positive charge in the order of 200 to 300 volts per metre near the earth's surface, though this can rise to as much as several thousand volts per metre depending on weather conditions. This electrostatic charge is created by extremely high energy cosmic rays as well as by the solar wind of sub-atomic particles and energies from the sun. The electrostatic nature of our atmosphere is an inherent aspect of weather conditions and it is not surprising that solar activity – solar flares and sun-spots etc – have an essential part to play in the earth's weather conditions. Thunderstorms are a releasing factor in this electrostatic potential gradient and are an integral part of the total, global picture.

Not surprisingly, this positive electrostatic field has a powerful effect on our life energies, together with the negative ions within our atmosphere. Plants sprout sooner and grow faster in a low energy electrostatic field and are disturbed by the absence of a field. More experimentation needs to be conducted, but it seems likely that similar effects will be observed to those noted from negative ionization of the atmosphere. The effect of the naturally occurring electrostatic Schuman waves have been discussed in the previous chapter.

In conventional science, a metal-mesh device known as a Faraday cage is used to shield out external electrostatic fields and, in a similar manner, many modern buildings have so much steel framework and wire cabling that the earth's natural field is severely distorted or altogether eliminated while you are inside. The subtle effect on our well-being must be present – yet another aspect of why we go outside 'to clear our heads'. Perhaps this is also one of the reasons why wooden buildings feel so good inside.

Geopathic Disturbances and Stress – Magnetic, Electromagnetic and Electrostatic

In addition to the earth's more obvious magnetic and electrostatic fields, there are also more subtle earth energies, detectable by direct intuition or subtle perception, as well as by dowsing. Dowsing (see chapter 10) is an ancient method, using a pendulum or other similar device, for detecting vibrations in subtle energy fields. It seems clear from dowsing evidence that there is a network of energy patterns and lines of force six or seven feet wide covering the surface of the earth. In fact, there would seem to be several levels of subtle energy of this kind, as one might expect. The Hartmann Net and Curry Grid are two that are the most frequently mentioned. This network is also connected with the ley lines of positive and negative energy that cross the earth's surface. The places where these energy strips cross have been called geopathic zones with associated symptoms of geopathic stress amongst people living in such places.

That animals are instinctively aware of these channels seems fairly clear. It is said for example that animal tracks often follow ley lines.

Underground water, as we discussed earlier, creates a negative energy above it and people living in dwellings built above such water often have health problems. Considerable research into the effect of underground water and geopathic zones has been made in Germany and Switzerland where the porous and fissured rock presents many such problem areas. Dr. Jenny, in a long series of tests between 1932 and 1945, observed the behaviour of mice kept in cages six metres long, partially over a zone of negative energy as detected by dowsing. Jenny noticed that four times as many mice nested away from the zone as within it and 13 per cent of mice confined to the zone, developed cancerous growths, the control groups remaining healthy.

Correlations between geopathic zones and scientifically understood energies are interesting though not always conclusive. J.W.F. Stangle, in 1973, reinvestigated the ground covered by two dowsers, Phol and Rambeau in the 1930's where they identified a higher incidence of cancer inside zones of negative earth energy, than without. Stangle also discovered that these zones contained a far higher level of background radio-activity than surrounding areas. Recent German studies have also linked slower blood clotting times to geopathic zones, as well as higher electrical conductivity (perhaps due to water content) in the earth itself.

One can draw no definite, 'scientific conclusions' from these facts except that they do fit in very well with other research findings concerning the existence of a powerful bio-electronic-magnetic organizing and informaton handling system within living creatures, that when disturbed, leads to illness.

Considerable work is still being done in West Germany and Switzerland on the effects, causes and types of geopathic and earth energies. This research is current and I present here a summary of their work to date, drawn mainly from the translations and writings of Anthony Scott-Morley, of the Institute of Bio-Energetic Medicine in Bournemouth, England.

Therapists and doctors of all callings are well aware that despite their best and most knowledgeable care, patients will respond very differently to treatment. This can be due to many factors, both within the patient and exteriorly in his environment. Amongst environmental factors must be considered the effect of subtle earth energies or *geopathic disturbances*. Quoting Scott-Morley:

'A geopathic stress may be defined as a *geomagnetic disturbance which is geographically localized and which disrupts the homeostatic mechanisms of the sensitive patient*. This definition should perhaps be widened to include man-made disturbances of an electrical, electromagnetic or radiation nature.

'Investigations by physicists and engineers have shown that geopathically disturbed zones exhibit a number of physically detectable characteristics.

'For example, there may be changes in the temperature gradient. Many buildings have 'cold' spots. There often appear to be cold draughts rising from precisely located spots which cannot always be accounted for by the proximity of doors and windows. (This phenomenon is often most easily observed in old churches, which were often built on energetically charged ground.)

'There can be a change in the degree of ionization due to electromagnetic field charges; AC charge also differs from the surrounding area. Electrical resistance changes, frequently being greater than the surrounding area.

There may also be changes in acoustic levels.

'Radio reception over a geopathically disturbed zone varies from that of the surrounding area; active gamma radiation is often detectable, and there is a measurable difference in the geomagnetic field.

'There are two broad categories of geopathic disturbance – the discharging field (yin), and the charging field (yang). These differences may be illustrated.

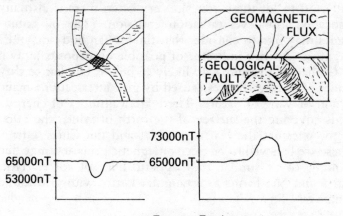

nT = nanoTessla
1 nT = 10⁻⁹ Tessla
1 Gauss = 10⁻⁴ Tessla

Discharging Field   *Charging Field*
Crossing point of two   *Geological fault zone*
underground streams.

'The height above ground level appears to make little or no difference to the intensity of these changes of flux intensity. Thus, a person living at the top of a tower block of flats is likely to be affected as much as the person at ground level.

'The discharging or yin forces are associated with the presence of underground water or underground caverns and hollows in the rock structure. Running water under pressure or hollows in the rock structure cause a decrease in the geomagnetic intensity which is often strong enough to influence the living organism. Where two underground streams cross, even though there may be many feet in vertical separation there is a greater geomagnetic disturbance. Surface water does not display this same phenomenon.

'Charging, or yang disturbances are more varied in nature, some emanating from geological phenomena and some arising from other sources. These disturbances are often associated with the presence of mineral deposits, especially coal and oil. The characteristics associated with the presence of oil deposits are changes in the degree of ionization; greater infra-red emission, AC and DC current changes; low frequency atmospheric pulsations (lightning will tend to hit these zones). Very often there is also an associated low level radiation emission. (The oil companies may like to consider that the human body may be the most sensitive indicator of possible oil deposits!).

'Global grid patterns are likely to be less familiar to the reader. The disturbances caused by grid intersections may be yin or yang in nature. There are a number of energy grids covering the surface of the earth of which the two major ones are the Hartmann Net and the Curry Grid. These are believed to be electromagnetic grids and may be thought of as similar to magnetic lines of force. The Hartmann Net forms a rectangular lattice with grid lines running N-S, E-W.

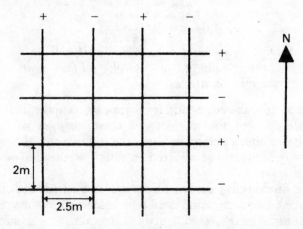

'*Schematic representation of the Hartmann Net: width of the grid lines is approximately 20 cm. Where the grid lines cross is an area of strong geopathic stress. Since the grid lines are 'charged' + or −, then if the intersection consists of two similar charges the disturbance is particularly noticeable. The width of the grid lines on the Hartmann net appears to increase to as much as 80 cm at*

the time of the full moon. Since the geopathic flux tends to be stronger at night-time when body resistance is weakest, the sleeping position of the patient is an important consideration. It is possible, for example, that the patient may have the head region of the bed within the area 80 cm × 80 cm but not in the area 20 cm × 20 cm. In this case symptoms would tend to be either seasonal or at the time of the full moon.

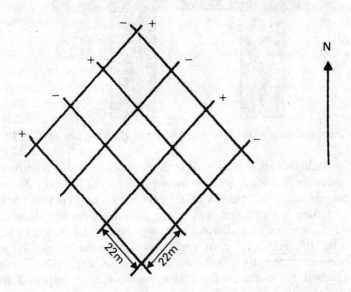

'*Schematic representation of the Curry Grid. This runs diagonally to the Hartmann Net. Note the change in dimension.*

'The Curry Grid is similar to the Hartmann Net except that it runs exactly diagonal to the Net and the distance between the grid lines is greater.

'The Curry Grid appears to be stable with respect to time and phase, ie the width of the grid lines does not vary.

'In both grids, the grid lines are charged alternately +, −, +, −. Where grid lines intersect with similar charges there is a strong geopathic disturbance.

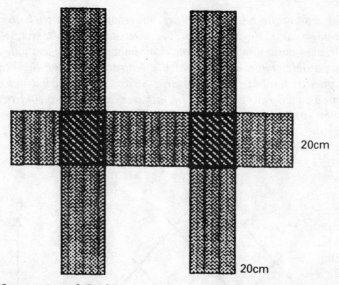

'Intersection of Grid Lines (Applies to Both Types of Grid)

'Radiation is another type of geopathic stress covering both corpuscular and non-corpuscular radiation. Non-corpuscular radiation is given off by certain types of rock structure (eg granite) and some mineral deposits such as oil. Corpuscular radiation is that given off by X-rays etc. With the latter type of radiation, the patient may have been exposed to excessive doses of X-ray; may have handled radio-active materials; or have been exposed to nuclear fall-out. The level of exposure to radiation needs to be only very slight (well below the 'safe' limit) to cause a disturbance in the sensitive patient.

'Electromagnetic fields from electrical apparatus may also be classified as geopathic in that they are energetic disturbances in the environment. Here we may think of the presence of electrical implements next to or close to the head, particularly while in bed (eg electrical clocks, radios); sleeping with an electric blanket switched on; current-carrying cables running behind the bed-head.

'Also to be considered are proximity to high voltage generators such as transformers and high voltage trans-mission lines such as those carried by electricity pylons.' (For an interesting case study, see the village of Fishpond in Dorset).

'If a cable carries an electric current then a magnetic field is generated. If the flux is strong and a person is within that field for lengthy periods of time, then the cellular mechanisms may become affected.

'Finally although not normally classified as geopathic stress, the practitioner should be aware of Schuman waves, which are a vertical radiation from the surface of the earth to the ionosphere. It seems that balanced health depends upon the presence of these waves. Unfortunately tall buildings and large expanses of concrete create an umbrella effect, blocking out the Schuman waves. Thus, large cities and towns tend to be deficient in Schuman waves with the consequent possibility of detrimental effects upon the inhabitants.

'The above examples cover the major geopathic forces which may stress the body. Undoubtedly, there are others which have yet to be discovered. Experienced practitioners who are aware of these stresses report that 30–50 percent of chronically sick patients exhibit some kind of geopathic stress of which the more common are the yin type stresses.

'It is probable that specific geographic locations have a higher incidence of geopathic stress than other areas.

Therapeutic Consequence of Geopathic Stress

'There is insufficient evidence to state that geopathic stress is the direct cause of disease. However, it does seem that geopathic stresses energetically weaken the body so that the patient may be more prone to disease-forming processes.

'The geopathic stress is an energetic force which, in the sensitive patient, is sufficiently strong to overcome the natural regulation and equilibrium of the body energy. Since it is the energetic equilibrium of the body which regulates and maintains the physiological well-being, if there is an overriding energetic dysfunction then physiological dysfunction must follow – the body can no longer maintain a homoeostatic balance.

'In the early stages, the patient frequently presents a non-specific and confused symptom picture. If the geopathic stress is not resolved the disease process will progress until a specific disease picture emerges. Any therapeutic intervention demands an energetic response from the body, but, because of the external stress, the body energy reserves are already being diverted and hence there is insufficient reserve left to respond to the therapeutic stimulus. Thus, the approved therapy often fails to work.

'The physiological effects of geopathic stress include: changes in the electrical polarity of the cell membrane, leading to impeded or faulty ionization across the cell wall; alteration of the spine oscillation and proton resonance of protein molecules; faulty hydrogen bonding; disturbances of the mesenchyme base regulation; disturbances of hormone balance; shifting of pH values; the promotion of vegetative disturbances.

Disease and Geopathic Stress

'There are a number of categories of disease which appear to be related to the presence of a geopathic burden on the body. It is thought that the geopathic stress may give a predisposition towards these disease states although we cannot claim that geopathic stress is the direct cause of these diseases.

Yin (Negative Stress)

'Hypo-, or energy deficiency disorders. E.g. fatigue; arthritis; cancer; multiple sclerosis; degenerative disorders. A negative field drains energy from the body leading to a deficient energetic state. It is thought that yin fields may be one of the main predisposing factors in malignant processes and degenerative disorders. There is also frequently a reversal of the spin oscillation of the protein molecules.

Yang (Positive Stress)

'Hyper-, or energy excess states. E.g. hypertension; cardiac problems including heart attacks; strokes; mania; alcoholism; migraine. Possibility of epileptiform fits in children. Yang fields lead to an excessive build up of energy in the body.

Grid Stresses

'Includes both of the above (Yin and Yang) depending upon the polarity of the grid intersection.

Radiation

'Skin complaints; fatigue. Long term effects of radiation burdening will lead to degenerative disorders. Radiation fields include both corpuscular and non-corpuscular types of radiation.

Electromagnetism

'Varied symptoms. Electromagnetic disturbances are often associated with mercury toxicity (arising from oral gal-vanic current formation between fillings). Thus one may expect to find symptoms associated with mercury toxic-ity, including central nervous system; renal; cardiac; and intestinal complaints. Electromagnetic disturbance is not only related to galvanic currents. Electrostatic sensitivity is also common. In these cases the patient may be sensitive to certain clothing fabrics, especially pure synthetic fabrics. It may be necessary to test for sensitivity to fabrics using small samples of suspect material. Very often the same material used in a mixture can be tolerated.

'Other sources of electromagnetic disturbance include battery operated wrist-watches; fluorescent lighting; bed-side electrical implements; microwaves; and VDU's as used in computers.

Detection of Geopathic Stress

'If carefully questioned, the patient will often describe symptoms which are frequently indicative of the presence of a geopathic stress. These include:

- Sleep disturbances; restless sleep; difficulty in getting to sleep
- Excessive dreaming
- Excessively heavy sleep but waking unrefreshed

- Excessive sleep requirements
- Cold legs and feet in bed
- Restless legs at night
- Respiratory difficulties at night. Asthma
- Excessive fatigue
- Unexplained mood changes; aggression; depression

'Children will often sleep on the edge of the bed or will curl up in one corner of the bed as though seeking to avoid the stressed area. They may be prone to sleep-walking and will often leave their own bed to climb in with their parents.

'It is interesting to note that many animals are sensitive to these stress forces. Dogs, goats, and cattle will always seek to avoid geopathically disturbed areas. When a dog moves round before lying down to sleep it may well be looking for the area of least disturbance. Cats, on the other hand, tend to seek out geopathically disturbed areas. If a cat has a favourite sleeping place (other than for reasons of warmth alone), it may well be that the place in question is geopathically disturbed.

'For the practitioner, it is important that the surgery be free from geopathic stress, especially the site of the treatment couch. If this area is stressed, then treatment results will often be poor and diagnostic information confused or misleading. Obviously, it behoves the practitioner to keep free from geopathic stress himself.

'When geopathic stress is suspected in the patient, it is important that this be dealt with before continuing further treatment. If the geopathic stress remains unresolved, the therapeutic results of normal treatment are likely to be less effective than would normally be expected. Frequently there is either little response to treatment, or there are unexpected relapses.

'The first suggestion to make is that the patient changes his/her sleeping position. The bed should be moved a few feet in one direction. If the stress is very localised (eg as from a grid stress), then this will often be sufficient to remove the patient from the influence of the stress. The body will often correct itself within three weeks of the effects of the stress. The patient reports sleeping better, feeling more relaxed and generally better in themselves.

'If a change of sleeping position produces no observable results, then further consideration has to be given. One possibility is to employ a skilled dowser to check the property of the patient and advise accordingly. A second (and often preferred) solution is to test the patient for specific geopathic stresses using bio-energetic tests such as the 'Vega' test. This will provide information concerning the type of stress affecting the patient. Depending on the nature of the stress, specific remedial measures can be taken although some detective work is often necessary. It may be for example that the patient is affected only by his work situation.

'Although removing the patient from the influence of the geopathic stress is both necessary and beneficial, it is sometimes found that this is insufficient. It is the author's experience that the geopathic stress often appears to get locked in the patient's body. The body appears to be incapable of rectifying the disturbance without further therapeutic measures. These specific measures depend on the nature of the stress and involve specialised use of homoeopathy and/or acupuncture. Since this is specialised treatment, it is not described in this article.

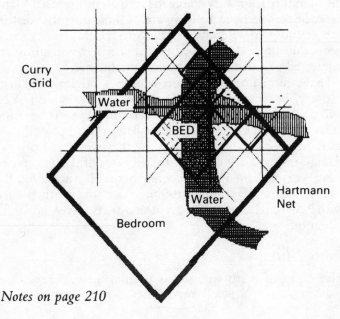

Notes on page 210

'This complex example shows an extreme possibility of geopathic stress. The bed is situated over a negative intersection of the Curry Grid which happens to coincide with a negative intersection of the Hartmann Net. Below the bedroom are two underground streams which cross. Thus, the bed is over an extremely yin geopathic area. Over a period of time, the occupant would have a high probability of developing cancer.

'The subject of geopathic stress is endlessly fascinating. It has great significance to the proper management of disease and yet comparatively little study has been made. It is suggested that there are many research possibilities in this subject. Yet, the subject and its significance is not entirely unknown. The effects of low energy changes on the body are suspected and have indeed been exploited by the military of both East and West. The most publicised experiment referring to these effects was shown on television when it was suggested that the USSR had been experimentally beaming low level/low frequency waves to the West ('Operation Woodpecker').

'Considering the amount of data available on the subject of geopathology, it is surprising that relatively little publicity has been given in this country. (This may be because most of the literature is only available in German or French.) Many practitioners seem to be unaware of these potential disturbances and even when aware often given little priority to the geopathic stress. It is hoped that this article will stimulate interested practitioners to investigate further.'

I have quoted Anthony Scott-Morley's article almost in its entirety, because of his understanding of the subject. You will no doubt have noticed many comments corroborating other ideas and experiences described in this book. Pulsor users in Switzerland have told me that while Pulsors can change the polarity of geopathically stressful areas, when there is a simultaneous intersection of the Hartmann Net, the Curry Grid and an underground water source, then even with Pulsors it is difficult to give the area a positive, healthful vibration.

Feng Shui

The study of earth energies is nothing new. There have been geomancers in all ages. The ancient Chinese art of

Feng Shui is probably the most detailed and intriguing way of channelling the flow of Ch'i in the environment. Indeed, although it is well known that the Chinese invented the first compass, it is not always made clear that it was originally designed as a geomantic aid, not for navigation. Clearly, the ancient Chinese understood the relevance of the earth's magnetic energies to harmonious living.

Shape and form are very important in the flow of energy. Energy flows upwards from the earth and out of corners and sharp edges. It also flows along and around certain shapes, thus explaining why certain hills and valleys have good atmospheres, while others feel dark and opressive. You will probably have noticed how simply closing the curtains will change the atmosphere in a room. The softness of the curtains obscures the view. Energy from the eye, too, can no longer travel into the wide open spaces, but is confined to a cosier environment. Energy from without can no longer penetrate within. A window without curtains looks bare, the curtains cover the effect of the sharp corners, which otherwise project negative energy into a room. Similarly, plants, which have a life energy of their own, can be draped over the edges and corners of bookshelves. Mirrors can be used to reflect and move energy in a confined space that would otherwise be blocked, stagnant or heavy. Wind-chimes are used, too, in Feng Shui, to break up concentrated flows of energy. In fact, many of the intuitive feelings and understanding of genuinely artistic architects, landscape designers, interior designers, sculptors and artists are within the understanding of Feng Shui. Think how different our landscape would be if all the ugliness of our man-made buildings and roads were subjected to planning permission based on the laws of Feng Shui or just good taste! The excuse that it would cost too much is not a good one either, for a good environment brings in good energy, one form of which is money. So money spent on good Feng Shui is an investment for all concerned. People would surely be more happy and productive in harmonious surroundings. Feng Shui literature abounds with stories of businessmen who have, for example, diverted their businesses from disaster by altering the entrance to their building to allow a more abundant flow of energy. Or they have changed the arrangement of furniture in their office or even closed off some of their abundant windows to prevent the energy and money from flowing right out again!

This is not as odd as it may sound upon first encounter. Everything, after all, is energy. When we perceive with our eyes, energy as electromagnetic vibration passes from the object to us carrying a representative pattern of the object encoded into that vibration or waveform. The eye focuses it, forms an inverted image of it on the retina, biochemically re-encodes the pattern as electrical energy and passes it down the optic nerve to the brain. After which nobody really knows what happens except that it winds up as vision, a faculty in which mental, emotional and subtle physical energies are also involved, the energy being transmuted through the vertical energy spectrum. So many of our energies are involved in 'simply' seeing things! And the quality of that energy will be an integral part of the way we go through life and the events that happen to us.

Feng Shui artists are employed in all areas of life, because everything is energy and its balanced flow is of paramount importance to our health, success, prosperity and beautiful environment. The rules of Feng Shui can determine the positive areas in the countryside, according to the shape of the hills and valleys and the presence of water in rivers, streams and lakes. Feng Shui can determine how to design roads and buildings, and where to position them. It can help choose a good site on which to live or run a business. It can influence the interior design and decoration of your house.

Money as Energy, Prosperity

The subject of money and prosperity is worth a brief digression, because it is a part of all our lives. As human beings, attachment, greed and insecurity are to a greater or lesser extent a natural part of our lot – something with which we all struggle. Attitudes towards money and business are as varied as people themselves and while some idealists may condemn the possession of money and property, due perhaps, to a subconscious knowledge of their own desires, others may wreck all chances of worldly success by an unconscious pseudo-spiritual, negativity, blocking their natural energy flow in fear of 'success' – perhaps because it does not fit in with the spiritual idea they have of themselves. Still others, quite genuinely, desire very little and are content with a simple life, while others strive all their life for money and possesions, with or without any success.

Money is energy – part of the surging pattern of our destiny. The acquisition of worldly riches, too, is more an attitude of mind than the fruit of hard work. Many a man has worked long hours for little recompense, while another always seems to be in the right place at the right time to make a 'killing'. Length of hours worked is not equatable to wordly fortune.

Money is like a river. It needs to flow to remain fresh and sweet. Even Christ looked askance at the man who simply buried his treasure, though Christ's meaning of 'treasure' may have been somewhat higher and spiritual. Energy, rightly used, can result in a healthly income. And a reasonable income can allow one to do many good things in life. A poor man, however good his intentions, cannot help another in his worldly fortunes, though he may have many other excellent human or spiritual qualities.

There is, in fact, a place for everyone and the possesion or non-possesion of riches is not a point for judgement of our fellow humans. It is important for our inner happiness, however, that our energy flows freely and easily, and this includes our relationship to money and the way we handle it. Prosperity means that we accept the good things of life, that we are a part of nature's abundance, that we do not dam up the river before it reaches us, nor attempt to hoard for ourselves everything that comes our way. Balance is required, as in all matters.

Money, or indeed any of our energies, should not be wasted. Neither should we waste the energies and money of other people through ill-considered or selfish activity or thinking. This is true from an ecological and planetary, as well as personal or moral point of view. Happiness and well-being will spring from a caring, thoughtful and focused use of the energies that pass before and through us.

Misappropriation of energy at any level will leave us ill at ease or miserable and will probably upset the mental and emotional balance of those misappropriated. Thus for example the thief, the manipulative businessmen as well as the manipulative customer, the emotionally attached and the greedy, all suffer from the same basic malady – mishandling of energy patterns. And they are all unhappy people, their degree of unhappiness being in relationship to the degree of imbalance in their mishandling of the natural law. This is our human situation.

With money perceived as just one of the energies that pass between us in our relationship with other humans, our approach to it takes on a different flavour. We will not take too much for services, neither will we take too little. Neither is there a standard amount that is applicable for all individuals to charge. It will depend upon where that money or energy flows after its receipt, in what energy complex of giving and receiving the receiver is placed. Many people judge others in this respect while only seeing the tip of the iceberg that relates to the full situation. We do not know the complete story of our own karmas, let alone those of others and are thus in no position to pass judgement, even within our own minds.

It is important too, that the energy or money we give should have no emotional strings attached that will tie us to the other individual or tie them to us. That is taking, not giving and the other person will consciously or unconsciously feel a drain of energy. Giving must be without thought of reward of any kind – material or emotional. If we give and have expectations and emotional involvement in some personally oriented outcome, we are not givers, however much we may fool ourselves concerning our 'generosity'.

All our relationships have a karmic origin. Our days are spent giving and receiving energy in one form or another. The wise man keeps these transactions of life balanced and clear, in accord with the natural law. He goes through life with as great a degree of consciousness, discrimination and balance as he can muster.

Energy involvements left unresolved in this life, need only to be cleared in another and it is thus through the muddiness and confusion of our day-to-day relationships that new karmas are created and we are kept forever on the wheel of reincarnation.

Pyramid Energies & the Influence of Shape

Knowing from a study of Feng Shui that shape is involved in the flow of energy, it is very clear that certain shapes will have special properties and it is not surprising therefore to find that shapes with a peak have good energy within them. Thus arches, domes, spires and pyramids, all have strong positive energy associated with their interiors. Dr. George Yao, the Pulsor creator, thinks that negative energy, *yin* in Chinese terminology, is drawn up and projected from the peak, leaving a balance of *yang*, or positive within.

In fact, it is well known that magnetic, electromagnetic or electrical energy are all projected or discharged from sharp points or corners. This is the principle behind lightning conductors, aerials (or antennae), as well as the corona discharge technique used in negative ion generators. Dr. Pat Flanagan discovered that the energy projected from the five corners of pyramids has the same properties as the energy within them which means that not all sharp-edge projected energy is negative. What all this does mean, however, is that conventional science does recognize the importance of shape and structure in an energy system, a thought not always applied to pyramid thinking.

What, after all, is shape? It is a change in the outward manifestation of vibrating energy patterns. Colours appear so, because the 'coloured' material is reflecting differing electromagnetic vibrations. Solids, liquids and gases take on form and structure according to the arrangement of molecules and atoms within them. Look around your immediate environment – the shapes of solids and air spaces appear so because of changes in the density and arrangement of their constituent molecules, atoms and sub-atomic particles. Shape and colour are entirely vibrational phenomena, so one would expect there to be some shapes with harmonious and some with disharmonious vibrations and atmospheres associated with them. This is a 'scientific' way of understanding Feng Shui, pyramid and other shape-related phenomena. Certain of the negative geomagnetic phenomena described are almost certainly related to the stresses, strains, shapes and disharmonies created at intersections and boundaries, while good earth atmospheres are no doubt attended by the harmonious arrangement of physical, as well as more subtle, structures.

The story of the modern day discovery of pyramid energies starts with the Frenchman, Bovis, in the late 1930's. While on holiday in Egypt and visiting the Great Pyramid of Gizeh, he was surprised to find a rubbish bin filled with small, dead animals, none of which showed signs of putrefaction. They were all simply dehydrated. One of the wardens told him that this was always the case with stray animals that got lost in the pyramid and ultimately died of starvation. When he returned home, Bovis began to experiment with model pyramids and obtained these same results.

When Bovis published his findings, one of his readers, Karel Drbal, a Czechoslovakian radio engineer, also became intrigued. During his experimentation, he discovered that if he kept his razor blade in the pyramid overnight, it was somehow sharp again in the morning. This was an important discovery, because good steel for razor blades was in short supply in communist countries. In fact, Russian soldiers were given only one blade a month, and that only lasted for a couple of shaves. Drbal had recalled his young army days, when the soldiers would, as a joke, put their friends razor blades on the window sill, so that the polarized moonlight would dull the edge without there being any visible signs of tampering.

Drbal's discovery was therefore of great practical value in his country, though it took him many years to persuade the patent's board to grant him a patent, he being unable to explain how his invention worked.

However the effect comes about, pyramids certainly generate energy that has both magnetic as well as subtle energy characteristics.

Some of the pyramid effects include the 'charging' of water, improvement of flavour in drinks and the dislike of micro-organisms and degenerative creatures like flies for the pyramid interiors. This latter is an interesting feature which is readily demonstrable because food stored in pyramids does not go rotten or mouldy, but has a tendency simply to dehydrate with age.

There is an interesting parallel here to our description of the tissue culture which was disturbed purely by the transmission of ultraviolet light from a bacterially contaminated culture. The ultraviolet, electromagnetic radiation is encoded with the negative, disharmonized vibration of the diseased culture and disturbs the uncontaminated culture by transmitting this vibration to its molecular and cellular structure. If we assume that there are positive and negative vibrations at the molecular, sub-atomic and subtle levels, as we discussed in previous chapters, then anything which is negatively attuned, such as degenerative micro-organisms, flies, etc., will find an area of positivity uncomfortable much as a violent and angry person will feel ill at ease in a spiritual community or a spiritual person feel out of place amongst disharmonious people. Hence, if the pyramid generates a positive energy vortex within itself, one can readily understand why the micro-organisms find no encouragement in their pursuit of rot and mould!

Similarly, with the improvement in taste, as well as the positive energy charging of water, affected by pyramids – something that can also be created by the use of Pulsors. Taste and the olfactory sense of smell are an appreciation of the molecular and atomic content of what passes through our mouth or nose. Flavour is improved not only by pyramids and Pulsors, but also by the mood of the cook. A woman who prepares food in a loving, concentrated state of mind will transmit this to all who partake of it, enhancing their consciousness and uniting all at the table in a spirit of warm communion, where no-one wants to leave and break the threads of harmony and good-will binding them. If, as we think, the olfactory sense also takes into account the molecular vibration and subtle energy content, in the same manner as the eyes seem to 'see' the aura, then we can readily understand how the flavour can be improved.

Interestingly enough, pyramids tend to remove or lessen artificial flavours and scents including those of sweets (or candies, if you are American) and cosmetics. They are left, respectively, with the sweet taste of sugar or that of the natural oil. The conclusion here would seem to be that the positive energy of the pyramid counteracts the un-natural vibrational quality in the artificial flavouring and scented molecules, relieving the molecules of their ability to stimulate the sensory cells.

Further evidence is also given to us by clairvoyants who tell us that prana is absorbed into the body through the back of the nose, while the vibrational healing element of flower essences takes place through the upper palate directly into the brain energy. It seems that the mouth and nose know a lot more about subtle energies than we might think on first taste!

The improvement in water quality can be explained along similar lines. Water or H_2O is, in any analysis, an odd substance. It expands when it solidifies, when most other materials contract. Without this one fact alone, the geological erosion of rocks by expanding ice in crevices would have given us quite a different-looking planet. Ice, therefore, is less dense and floats, hence we have ice-bergs, pack-ice and so on. In fact, the entire north pole and arctic circle would be quite different if ice sank! The forms of H_2O such as hail, snow and rain, plus its affinity to so many other molecules all add up to its being a unique substance with many other more abstruse properties we don't have space for here. Some scientists, for example, think that water actually has crystalline properties, oscillating in and out of the solid state many times per millisecond, thus maintaining the properties of a liquid. Water also has a di-pole molecule. That is to say that, electrically speaking, its charge is not equally distributed over its surface, but is polarized: positive at one end, and negative at the other. This means that it is affected by regular magnetism and this factor has been used by therapists for many years. 'Magnetized' water has been used by Ayurvedic medicine for centuries and magnetism we know is very close in vibrational frequency to the more subtle energies, producing effects at those levels, as evidenced by the ability to stimulate acupuncture points with small magnets.

Water, too, being the universal solvent in which physical life processes take place would need to be a carrier of pranic and subtle energies in order to fulfil its function.

Tap water left in pyramids (or treated by Pulsors) loses some of its chlorine flavour, tastes better, is said to have healing properties, makes plants grow better and faster and is preferred by (probably nine out of ten!) dogs and cats. It also holds its subtle energy charge longer that other substances, such as bread and foodstuffs. Pyramid treated foods do last two or three times longer than untreated foods, but the rot does set in sooner or later.

There is an interesting relationship of crystals to pyramid energy. Dr. William Tiller of Stanford University has used standard laboratory techniques for growing crystals under pyramids. Some of the odd effects he reports include crystals with spiral and striated distortions as well as those with peculiar optical and piezo-electric properties.

Other properties of pyramids include the creation of a weak magnetic field, even in those made of cardboard, that pyramids work best with one side aligned to magnetic north and that pyramid effects can vary from day to day, perhaps due to variations in the earth's magnetic field and most probably to the variations in subtle energy quality and quantity in the vicinity of the pyramid. In this context, it would be interesting to know if the effect of pyramids varies according to where they are and who is using them. Again, we find an association of magnetism with subtle energies. We should point out that science does not know what magnetism, or indeed any matter or energy actually *is*. It only describes properties and relationships. And until the understanding dawns concerning the vertical energy spectrum, conventional science will always be beating its head against a wall. The facts will never add up. And once this is understood, then one realizes that nothing can ever be *explained*, only *described*. *Explanation* or *understanding* come only from inner experience – totally subjective and therefore, of course, a matter of grave suspicion to the 'objective' scientist. C'est la vie!

Using bio-feedback equipment to monitor the voltages, pyramids seem to affect the brain waves towards relaxation, of those sitting, meditating or sleeping in them. We have never done any experiments with brain-wave measurement and Pulsors, nor heard of anyone doing any, though the deep relaxation experienced must be reflected in the brain waves. Many of the subjective comments we hear from people are very similar. With an open frame pyramid over the bed, people report sleeping less, feeling more refreshed on waking and being more alert and energetic during the day, while dreams are often more vivid, colourful and memorable.

Subtle and psychic awareness is also enhanced – people say they see lights and colours within their body and certain kinds of meditative states are deepened, with a corresponding reflection in the amplitude of the alpha brain waves.

CHAPTER 9

The Etheric or Health Aura

The Etheric Body

Throughout this book, I have attempted to avoid the word etheric, not because of any personal dislike, but because it has been used so much and so variously that it means different things to different people and induces differing responses, too. The etheric body or etheric double was first described in detail and in print to the western world by the Theosophists, although we could not attribute its *discovery* to them. Psychically gifted people, yogis and mystics throughout all ages and cultures have been aware of it, as is evidenced from their writings and paintings. The oriental writings of India, Tibet and China are full of descriptions of

Comprised of the subtle forms of the five tattwas, the etheric body lies within the physical frame, extending a few inches away from the physical body as the health or etheric aura. Within its many energies and ramifications are contained the chakras and nadis, as well as the acupuncture meridians and the life-giving, vibrational patterning of the pranas. It represents the immediate blueprint of our bioelectronic energy system as well as the observable solid, fluid, gaseous and calorific (heat) aspects of our physical body. It is the transmitter and receiver of higher emotional and mental energies from above and physical energies from below. That it has higher and lower levels of energy within it, is evidenced by the fact that although many people can see this aura as an interplay of colours, very few are able to see deeper or higher to perceive the chakras or the flow of energy in the acupuncture meridians and fewer still can read it consistently and correctly for the identification of health and disease problems within the physical organism.

It is from within this etheric matrix that energy is distributed to the physical body. Here we find the close connection of the endocrine glands with the chakras as controlling centres of energy. There are also many minor plexi, crossroads or control points for energy flow, just as the physical brain or heart tissues have a more central organizing role to play than, for example, the muscles of the leg. Hence, psychics and therapists have described the spleen and its etheric counterpart as a storer and distributor of subtle energy throughout the gross physical and etheric bodies.

The etheric body has also been described as a web-like structure with some bodies being closely knit and others torn or fragmented. The expression being 'spaced out', for example, used by habitual drug abusers indicates exactly what has taken place in their etheric body, where their integrity and shape has received a violent rending and the energy flow has been disrupted so that continuity, concentration and co-ordination of thoughts and physical actions becomes difficult. Such is the case, too, with alcohol. Many people who meditate spontaneously give up the use of drugs, alcohol, coffee and even tea because of the disruptive effect on their inner state of being, to which they have developed a heightened sensitivity.

Miasms and The Vibrational Pattern of Disease

During the latter part of the eighteenth and the early years of the nineteeth century, the German physician Samuel Hahnemann (1755–1843) researched and established the principles of what he termed homoeopathy. Seeking to treat the whole person, homoeopathy provides remedies which establish vibrational harmony within the subtle energy fields of our physical being. The different remedies, with their differing vibrational characteristics, are matched to the treatment of the different disharmonies that are present in all of us.

Hahnemann, however, took this principle further. There are, he felt, certain basic vibrational patterns of disease, which he termed *miasms*. Miasms originate in the subtle or auric field setting up 'patterns' in an individual's life and body. Like a drop of dye in a bucket of water, or like a pinch of salt in a stew, these vibrations or miasms spread their subtle influence throughout *all* the energies of our being. Miasms, said Hahnemann, are acquired – by various contagions or from traumatic influences experienced during the course of our lives – and manifest through the established vibrational outflow of sub-atomic, atomic, molecular, electromagnetic and general biochemical and physiological processes in our bodies.

Depending upon the intensity of the miasmatic vibration these patterns may be either inherited genetically or acquired by resonance – 'we are influenced by the company we keep' says the old saying. Indeed it is truer and deeper than we may imagine. Miasms may therefore be acquired during a lifetime or derived from parents before birth. Inherited miasms will be transmitted through the genetic code – the cellular intelligence and memory – whilst acquired influences reflect as or may be caused by bacterial or viral attack or, in modern times, by levels of toxic pollution in our food and environment.

Some schools of thought also talk about planetary miasms, that is to say subtle tendencies and vibrations within the mood or collective unconscious and subtle energy of the planet itself. These can also be disturbed and changed by the care, or lack of it, administered by the inhabitants. Pollution and rape of the environment thus cause planetary disharmonies at both subtle and gross levels which disturb the health of all creatures living here. Simon Martin had some interesting comments to make along these lines in his foreword.

Miasms may also lie dormant in an individual for many years manifesting only in subtle ways until such time as the person is weakened by external or internal causes. These tendencies will then flare up causing illness, stress, biological degeneration of the tissues, loss of vitality and old age. The subtle energy patterns then exhibit themselves more openly in the weakened person at the biochemical and physiological level or they may become evident as bacterial or viral infections which have lain dormant or in symbiotic relationship, then multiplying at the expense of their host, the natural vibrant resistance to disease being severely curtailed.

Miasms spread throughout the mental, emotional and subtle physical or etheric energies of our constitution and represent a part of the pathway by which the karmas of actions and tendencies of previous lives manifest as ill-health in our present life.

Energy is never lost, only transformed or relocated and homoeopathic cure attempts, therefore, to smooth out the disharmony of the miasm, as the basic cause of disease, thereby treating the whole person. The release of the entire miasmatic trait would result in a complete cure, more or less impossible in totality since the higher energy constituting the karmic origin of our existence on this plane ensures that perfection in the energy patterns of our mind–emotion–body complex can never be attained. Perfection is, however, obtainable in soul regions, whilst the human aspects still live out their karmic destiny. If therefore, a miasm is successfully treated, the energy field is re-polarized, but the person still retains the tendency to live out the same pattern.

Miasms are essentially an energy disharmony, dis–ease pattern or imbalance. It is not necessary, therefore, to *remove* the energy but only to *rearrange* the energy patterns into a more harmonious nature, just as a storm is a vibrational disturbance that once abated, leaves the surface of the same water clear and calm.

Hahnemann spoke of three major inherited miasms: *psora*, *sycosis* (gonorrhea) and *syphilis*. Psora is deficiency or imbalance, per se. A keyword to describe it is irritation. Thus it manifests as skin eruptions of all kinds, as disharmony of the body's natural rhythms, and emotionally as tiredness, depression, worry, timidity, anxiety and fear. Hahnemann felt that psora, being imbalance, was the essence or mother of all disease, leading to the other two miasmatic traits.

The *sycotic* miasm is represented by excess, exuberance, hyper-function, and over-activity, the word itself coming from the Greek, meaning 'wart' or 'excrescence'. It expresses itself as hyper-activity in all the major organs and systems of the body. Digestive, respiratory, cardio-vascular and urinary problems abound, characterized by discharges, whilst overheated mental and emotional activity result in a harried, extrovert, ambitious and ostentatious nature, that can even lead in extreme cases to psychiatric and clinically psychotic conditions.

The *syphilitic* miasm is degenerative and destructive in its effect. People in whom this miasm is strong are easily disturbed and have cruel and destructive aspects to their nature, their physical diseases are characterized by ulceration, erosion and tissue decay.

The terms used by Hahnemann reflected the problems and diseases of his time in history, but looked at from a more universal point of view, we can see very clearly the duality or polarity that he is attempting to express. The syphilitic miasm is an expression of the Indian tamas guna or the yin of the Chinese. It is winter, death, inertia, darkness and neglect.

The sycotic miasm, on the other hand, is a manifestation of the outgoing, active, rajas guna or yang principle. It is expression, manifestation, activity, positive. Psora represents a state of imbalance (viz. a deviation from 'central integrity' or Tao), whilst health, as Hahnemann so astutely observed, comes from eliminating this disharmony or psora.

So we are back once again with the essential principles of polarity and duality, expressed in Western idiom.

Some schools of thought have considered whether tuberculosis or cancer are true miasms and more recently it is said that there are three new miasms coming into existence from the high levels of environmental pollution. These are the petrochemical, the radiation and the heavy metal miasms. There is no doubt that tuberculosis and pollution hazards manifest with specific identifiable symptoms, causing particular kinds of subtle and gross disharmonies that are identifiable as unbalanced vibratory patterns and could hence be termed miasms. They can, however, still be understood in terms of the essential duality of nature and are really only a sub-aspect of this reality. They can still be expressed in terms of psora, syphilitic and sycotic miasms, as rajas, tamas and satvas gunas or as the yin and yang of the Chinese. This does not of course, make them any the less serious – it just gives us the underlying understanding of what is taking place and how Hahnemann's doctrine of the three miasms holds good even in the present day.

In this respect, it is interesting to see how Chinese herbal medicine, for example, administers herbs with a knowlege of their yin and yang characteristics and effects, while Islamic traditional medicine talks similarly of their 'hot' and 'cold' aspects. They are thus used with a similar intent to homoeopathic remedies – to balance the basic energies that constitute our human existence. But oriental herbal systems aim to counteract the hot or cold imbalance whereas homoeopathy seeks to match the total symptom picture of the patient with the total symptom-producing picture of the most similar remedy.

It is possible that Hahnemann was not seeking such a fundamental approach to the basis of disease as I have suggested by equating the miasms with the inherent duality in the universe. In that case, one can simply consider the miasms as ubiquitous subtle vibrations within the human energy system, behind and within which lie the basic driving forces of polarity imbalance and disharmony. No human being has ever encapsulated the whole of a science within their life's work and it is certain that such an advanced thinker as Hahnemann would have continued with the evolution of his understanding and practice had he continued to live until the present day! The tendency of human beings to crystallize their thinking around the work of an expert long-departed – whether in the field of religion or science – points not so much to the infallibility of the departed hero as to the lack of truly original thinkers and barrier-breakers amongst us.

In fact, it is said from various psychic and similar sources that homoeopathy itself is not new and that similar potentized energy medicines were used both in Atlantis – where crystal resonance was used for energizing medications – and Lemuria, where the subtle essence was derived from plants, perhaps in a similar manner to that used in the preparation of the modern Bach flower remedies.

The truth of the environmental conditions causing the new vibrational patterns has been frequently mentioned throughout this book. Environmental pollution must be countered if we are to survive with anything like our existing social structure, civilization and technology into the twenty-first century. Man must bring his technology into harmony with nature, for this is our only hope. Everyone has a personal responsibility to resist his own tendencies towards self-interest and personal profit in order that the planet remains a reasonably decent place for others to inhabit. If people only realized the inexorable nature of the law of karma, of cause and effect, spanning across all our lifetimes, then even out of selfish motives, nobody would create such dirty messes in this world. They would know that they will be re-born to feel the effect of their previous wanton destruction of the earth!

Relating to our discussion of miasms, a hypothesis put forward by Dr. J.E.R. McDonaugh, is that viruses are created by the dis-harmonious vibration (he calls it over-expansion) of protein molecules, causing pieces to break off, becoming the virus. This virus then goes rogue through the normal processes of protein reproduction and can infect other healthy organisms. Many holistic practitioners would add that the disease can only take root if there is a propensity for it – a vibration within the organism, with which the negative nature of the disease can resonate, in other words, a miasm.

This *vibrational pattern* aspect of disease or ill-being occurs at all levels. A negative thought or idea fed to us from without cannot affect us unless it finds some corner – greater or lesser – with which it can resonate. Neither can an illness, even an epidemic, affect us, unless there is a vibrational seed in us, by which its entrance may be effected, through sympathetic resonance. In this way, we attract things to ourselves, both good and ill. In karmic terms, if we are destined through actions or thoughts in past lives to reap the result in this life, then that pattern will be an inherent part of our constitution from the moment of our birth – either mentally, emotionally or physically – and will come to fruition at the right time, in the right place and in the right way. This is the manner of the outworking of our destiny for good, bad or indifferent and large or small events in our life. *But*, say the sages, *we have a conditioned free-will*, within the context of our destiny, within which we have the capacity to create new karmas for future lives either good, bad or middling! We are not absolutely free, but are governed by the energy patterns recorded in higher energies as on a wax tablet, which determine the main structure and much of the detail in our present life. Thus, as long as we are separate from the One Ocean and have a separate sense of identity or ego, then we must use our discrimination to make correct decisions about our activities and the thoughts we entertain. In as far as one realizes that one's life is not in one's own hands and the little 'I' simply does not exist, then one can surrender to the great Omniwill.

Emotional and Mental Energies and Their Presence Within the Aura

As we discussed in previous chapters, emotional and mental energies are a higher vibration than the subtle physical energies. In some schools of thinking, they are included within the etheric body, in others they are equated with the astral and causal bodies. However, the real astral and causal bodies, operating in their respective worlds, are higher up, more inward, as previously described. For myself, I think of these emotional and mental energies as subtle energies within the body and a part of the continuum or spectrum of energies. In terms of the aura, these energies certainly have a larger 'spread' than the purely subtle physical or etheric aura, as can be demonstrated with dowsing rods or by one's own intuitive experience. The presence of a person in a room can be clearly felt at both a physical, emotional and mental level. Sexual attraction normally occurs when physically very close to someone. Certainly one is more affected by another person's vibration when sitting next to them. But the emotional and mental content of another person's mind is spread throughout a house. The feeling of being totally alone in a house is common to many people, as is the knowledge of another's presence, without any noises or other clues to their being there.

The associations we have with individuals provide us, too, with a link. Even over oceans and continents, space appears to be no barrier. The inward and the outward are very close, more so than conventional science would care to think.

In fact, the aura is an expression of the soul within and its surrounding bodies and energies. The physical, astral and causal bodies are integrally linked with their emanating energies in the aura, reflecting the nature of the being within. Imagine how glorious must be the aura and appearance of a saint, sparkling with the light of love and mystic wisdom. Compare it with the low, dull, coarseness of an angry, depraved and cruel person. For the latter, you feel sadness, but turn away because there is little or nothing you can do; but the saint you could gaze at forever and never feel satiated.

Charisma

Also known as personal magnetism, charisma is a quality of attraction that surrounds some individuals. Often associated with a high level of inexhaustible physical energy and endurance, charismatic people become the centre of attention wherever they go. Frequently they are leaders or entertainers. People find it stimulating and energising to be in their presence, especially if the nature of their personality is akin to one's own.

Politicians, great generals, philosophical leaders all have this quality in common. One thinks of the great Alexander who during the early years of his life led his army on the long journey from Persia to India, holding his territories under control even from far afield, without modern means of communication, through the love and respect, and also fear, created by his personality. Hitler too, had a charisma and magnetism that drew people to him in unthinking loyalty. He had personal charm, as well as a demoniacal aspect. All such leaders must have this quality in order for them to hold their position for any period of time. And it is not necessarily equated with goodness or spirituality.

Charisma in entertainers is more or less a prerequisite: a subtle means of reaching out and touching the hearts of their audience. Amongst true spiritual teachers or mystics, charisma is an inherent, outward manifestation of their inward and loving being. Indeed, charisma associated with a spiritual tendency makes for an extremely charming personality. However, it should not be mistaken for spirituality – a likeable, powerful and magnetic personality is not equatable with inner spiritual knowledge. Charisma is seen in the aura as a strong and energetic vibration at etheric, emotional and mental levels. It is also the 'joie de vivre'. The Chinese say that such a person has strong Ch'i. Definitely, such people have an abundance of being in their outward manifestation, that can exert a powerful influence over others.

CHAPTER 10

Dowsing and the Detection of Subtle Energies

Pendulums and Divining Rods

Dowsing, divining or radiesthesia is the art of detecting energies, objects and so on, by means of special rods, pendulums or instruments, an essential component of all such methods being the operator himself, without which nothing happens. The dowsing literature is replete with historical references to water divining, probably the oldest known form of dowsing. There are numerous works of art and paintings throughout the ages of all cultures depicting water diviners at work, the earliest known of which is possibly a statue of the Chinese Emperor Kwang Su, dated at around 2200 BC, holding a forked twig divining rod.

In recent centuries, and probably earlier too, dowsing rods and pendulums were used for locating minerals, as well as water, and since the early part of the twentieth century, dowsing instruments have been used for medical and subtle energy detection applications (radionics and radiesthesia). Since there is rarely anything new amongst natural phenomena, I would not be at all surprised if medical radiesthesia and all forms of dowsing were used by people of older cultures. It is only our modern mania, backed up by technology, for the high-speed printed word and writing things down, that has laid out everything in black and white for all ages to know. In previous ages, knowledge was largely transmitted by word of mouth, from teacher to pupil, often in secrecy. Sometimes, indeed, this passion for secrecy was so strong that ultimately, the knowledge died with its holders. This is true, for example, of ancient China where families would develop special knowledge of acupuncture that made them famous and, no doubt provided a healthy income. But when ultimately, the family died out, this knowledge was lost with them.

It is not my intention to array the evidence for the dowsing phenomenon here. This has been done in many other books. Suffice it to say that most armies of the world, most mineral, mining, water and pipe-line companies and many farmers and builders in dry areas all have dowsers on their payroll or employ them from time to time. Such people don't use dowsers unless it works.

Moreover, dowsing has historically been and is being used increasingly in therapeutic practice, mostly within so-called Alternative Medicine, with great success, in diagnosing both physiological and biochemical disturbances and deficiencies as well as the subtle energy condition of the patient.

Dowsing has also been employed to find submarines (using a map) and mines, map the aura, check the sex of day-old chicks (in Japan), find criminals in hiding (again using a map), decide which car to buy or which dress to wear, finding lost articles, perform remote radionic and Pulsor diagnosis and treatment, discover the sex of your unborn baby, find or date archaeological discoveries, and much, much more. If you have never had a go, it is worth trying. You can make rough divining rods out of wire coat-hangers and anything small, heavy and symmetrical will make a pendulum to start off with. It's good fun and many people have the natural talent, which normally grows with practice and experience, so don't be afraid of being thought a nutcase!

For those who do not know anything concerning dowsing, perhaps some brief description will be of help. First of all, a dowsing instrument is required. Some of the commonest are illustrated overleaf.

To successfully use any dowsing instrument, you need to understand clearly what is happening. Firstly, *the real detector is yourself* – your own bio-energy field, your subconscious and perhaps even your superconscious, mind. There is a part of us that knows everything, but we are not consciously in contact with that part. Or perhaps it is as simple as the fact that although I can raise my hand, I do not know *how the thought is transferred* from my mind to the brain, to the nerves, to the muscles and to the contractile muscle cells. So if all the basic aspects of having a body and

A.

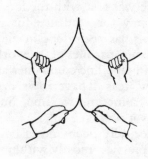

Traditional water divining rod about 12″ long, made in wood (often hazel or willow), also metal, plastic, whalebone, etc., held in the hands with palms uppermost. It dips down or up when the dowser passes over whatever it is they are dowsing for. Small ones, about 6″ long, held in the fingers are also used sometimes.

B.

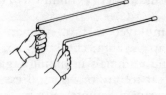

Dowsing rods, about 12″ long, of the kind often used for aura mapping. They are held horizontally, parallel and pointing forward, one in each hand. They cross over or move apart when the energy field is detected. The handle is a tube in which the L-shaped rod can swivel.

C.

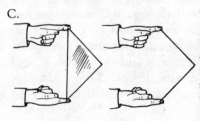

Triangular shaped either in plastic or a metal wire, about 6″–8″ high, the apex of the triangle points forward and moves to one side or the other when whatever it is, is detected.

D.

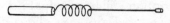

This is a design first used by the famous American dowser the Reverend Verne Cameron, for aura mapping. It moves to one side or the other upon detection.

E.

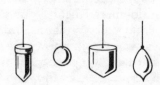

Various shapes and sizes of pendulum, made of all manner of materials. The direction of swing indicates the answer to the question or the presence of an energy field. The string is normally about six inches long, though it can be much longer when used with some special techniques.

how it works are a mystery to our conscious mind, then perhaps we can accept that our bio-energy system 'knows' more than we do about certain things?

So *we* are the detector – the dowsing instrument is simply like the needle on an electronic meter. It *indicates* what we unconsciously already know or detect. Therefore, it is necessary for the dowser to be very clear in his or her mind what they are looking for. Learning to maintain the *correct attitude* and *clarity of intention* is most of the problem in learning to dowse successfully, representing the major cause of inaccuracies and errors. This also means that if you are upset or emotional, your unbalanced energies will result in unreliable readings. Calmness and concentration are required. You can do this by mentally or verbally asking a question, e.g. is there underground water here? Or by simply holding one's intention in mind. If you are dowsing for water then you can think of a waterfall, or a flowing river, or the sea – anything that tunes you into water, while at the same time holding in mind that that is what you are seeking. If monitoring earth energies and ley lines, you can keep an image of rock or volcanoes in mind, or simply tune in to the *feeling* of the energies sought after.

The success of dowsing depends upon the degree to which you can detach yourself from the result or the answer, while at the same time maintaining a caring, disinterested interest in the outcome. If you try too hard to be 'fair' and not to influence it, you will kill it stone dead. If you have a strong conscious or subconscious desire or predjudice for the outcome to be one way or another, you will probably influence the pendulum or dowsing rods. You need to develop a high degree of personal integrity and honesty to be able to use a dowsing instrument successfully. I always tell my wife, for example, that there is no use in using her pendulum, when trying to decide whether or not to buy a dress she likes. The pendulum will have an inherent tendency to say 'yes'!

Some dowsers have different instruments for different purposes, because that helps to keep their mind clear as to what they are dowsing for – water, earth energies, minerals or aspects of the aura and so on. Some dowsing rods have a section in the handle to place a specimen of what is being sought – it is known as a witness. This helps to channel the mind of the user towards that substance. It can even be a piece of paper with a particular key name or word written on it. The witness helps the user to make a mental commitment towards seeking that thing. It is also probable that the vibration of the witness helps the user to attune to the vibration of what is being sought. There are pendulums, too, with spaces within them for a witness.

Having said all this about honesty and tuning in, it is still likely or possible that you will make errors. Even the great Reverend Verne Cameron, who in 1959 successfully located on a map, all the United States submarines before the surprised gaze of Vice Admiral Curtis and followed it up by pinpointing all the Russian submarines, 'discovered' in his aura mapping that auras had angelic wings and halos. His Christian background found an aura not confirmed by any other dowsers or psychics! Verne Cameron does give some good advice when he suggests visualizing the dowsing instrument as an extension of your own body, complete with nervous and muscular connections.

The material of which the instrument is made may also have an effect upon the accuracy and use of the pendulum. Perhaps a steel pendulum or dowsing rod would be best for detecting magnetism and earth energies, while copper would be appropriate for seeking out electrical cables and induction fields. Crystal pendulums may be of help in zeroing in on specific healing colours or aspects.

Since dowsing is clearly connected with the bioelectronic and subtle energy fields, which have activity in magnetic and electromagnetic/biomagnetic energy fields, it is probably wise to avoid metal and electrically conductive pendulums when dowsing for the state of subtle energies. Similarly, the thread can be of cotton or silk, with nylon perhaps being suspect because of its electrostatic properties. Subtle energies definitely 'pass' along wires, in channels, and over natural dividing lines as is evidenced by psychic perceptions, the nadis and acupuncture meridians, while shapes have an influence too, as we know from the pyramids and Feng Shui. What is required is a device that will not block or disturb the flow of your energies, so if you do not like a particular material or dowsing instrument, then don't use it.

We always use a Pulsor pendulum, the Acu-Pulsor, when working with Pulsors and detecting these levels of body energy polarities, because other pendulums can have mixed subtle energy polarities and can cause inaccurate readings. Even generally, we find the Acu-Pulsor to be highly accurate and reliable.

Some people do not like their dowsing instruments to be touched by others, since this disturbs their vibrations. This is quite understandable. The essential point is that whatever helps you to be clear of intention and honest in your use should be adopted.

With all of the devices pictured, the user needs therefore to determine within himself what are the positive and negative responses of his chosen device. Will the divining rod (A) go up or down, for example, to indicate water or minerals? Will the rods (B) open out or cross over? Does left or right indicate a 'find' with the triangular shapes (C) and the Cameron Aurameter (D)?

The pendulum offers a three-choice situation:

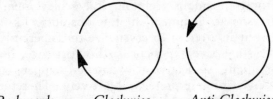

Forwards/Backwards   *Clockwise*   *Anti-Clockwise*

Depending upon what you are detecting, you can programme your response to be either two or all three of these options. The amount of movement is normally taken to mean the strength of the field or the 'yes' or 'no' response. To programme your response you simply tell yourself very clearly which is the positive and which the negative and whether gradations in between, relating to the extent of the movement, are meaningful to you. And then stick to it, so that it becomes second nature.

Practice and association with other dowsers will help to bring out your latent talents. Sometimes a reluctant pendulum or divining rod will spring to life just by the presence of an expert or when he puts his hand on yours.

It is difficult to provide a rational and scientific explanation of how and why a pendulum works. However, work it does and my own feeling is that the pendulum uses the body's own bio-energy to represent in clockwise or anti-clockwise motion the polarities or state of harmony of whatever is being tested. The subtle, etheric forces of nature require a subtle test and measurement device that in this case draws on the human operator for its source of power. For this reason, it is essential that the human operator is correctly balanced. An incorrectly balanced operator will get confusing and misleading results – this is indeed the experience of many dowsers to whom we have spoken. The use of Pulsors, or some similar method, for calibrating a pendulum and checking on one's own polarities and state of harmony is therefore a pre-requisite for accurate readings of subtle energies.

While standard, scientific methodology requires so-called objective, empirical test and measurement verification, we should bear in mind that this way of thinking is just a mode of thought, prevalent historically, for only a short space of time. And while it has been responsible for tremendous technological achievement, there is no reason to assume that it is absolute. Its validity stems from an attempt to crystallize the inherently fluid aspects of subjective experience. All experience, however, is essentially subjective – whatever happens to us is perceived or interpreted subjectively. Therefore, to require an empirical, objective verification of experience before it is considered as valid, is to reduce the power of life, love and consciousness to its lowest common denominator and to rob it of its power of intercourse with physical matter.

It is said that we are entering a New Age, astrologers call it the Aquarian Age. The technology of this New Era will require an interaction of the individual with his devices in a subjective yet higher scientific manner. The natural tendency of humans to mistrust each other, because of separation from and lack of knowledge of each other, needs to be transmuted, so that we understand with love, the failings and strengths of our fellow creatures and are able to find the point of balance and discrimination in subjective, scientific study. Intuition needs to become an accepted and valid aspect of research and technology.

Getting Started

A suitable pendulum can be made out of almost any small object by hanging it on about four to six inches of thin cotton or chain. According to Dr Yao, crystal pendulums should be used with caution since they have polarity problems of their own and can give incorrect readings. A crystal pendulum should be cut on the C-axis (light axis) and leaded crystal glass should not be used since the transmitted light can cause polarity reversals in the body.

To accurately dowse for subtle energies, you must be as free from subtle energy reversals and disharmonies as possible. So firstly, remove all metalwork and cigarettes or other negative items from your person and sit or stand without crossing your arms or legs and with your feet flat on the floor. This allows your energies to move in a harmonious manner and in good contact with the earth.

Then move away from electrical applicances, fluorescent lights, metal furniture or radiators for a distance of at least four to six feet. This takes you out of the immediate vicinity of any normal electric fields.

Now, holding the pendulum in your right hand, between the thumb and the forefinger, swing it freely to and fro, mentally asking a question of your own unconscious knowledge.

Observe the result with a relaxed and detached mind. The pendulum is easily affected by your own mind in its direction of rotation, but the technique of a loving, detached, observation should be inculcated. A forced mental attempt *not* to influence the pendulum will also affect it, often resulting in its refusal to move at all! The shoulder, wrist and forearm muscles should be relaxed. A stiff wrist will also kill the motion of the pendulum.

Dowsing is a skill which can be learnt and which develops with practice. Association with an experienced dowser is also most helpful in getting your own skill going. If you have problems, check your surroundings for obviously negative influences, try moving a few feet away from other people, or changing your clothes to light coloured and natural fibres. Or try facing south or any other direction which helps to make it work.

How Does Dowsing Work?

A pendulum or dowsing rod moves because the dowser involuntarily moves it. Occasionally, the muscular contraction with forked twig dowsing rods is enough to break them. You can perform an experiment with yourself by holding a pendulum and mentally telling it to move clockwise or anti-clockwise. If you had a video camera trained on your fingers, you would actually see them moving. With dowsing rods, the muscular contractions of the hands and forearms are immediately apparent. This, perhaps immediately damns the whole thing in the eyes of the sceptic, but the question is, why do the muscles move? Moscow and Leningrad Universities both have departments devoted to researching *how* (not *if*) dowsing works. The immediate scientific approach has always been to see if it is electromagnetic or magnetic in nature. Dowsers can, after all, detect very weak magnetic fields one two-hundredths of the earth's field, can know if an electrical device is switched on or off and can locate the sources of radio and TV broadcasting. There is iron in haemoglobin, or water in our tissues, with magnetic properties, reason some researchers. Well, shielding dowsers in lead and similar enclosures that block the transmission of electromagnetic and magnetic fields, does not stop their abilities any more than it does telepathy.

My own feeling is that at whatever level you are seeking knowledge of an energy field, at that level the unconscious mind or body energy reaches out, knows the answer and automatically taps it in to our vertical energy spectrum, and out it comes through the reflex contraction of certain muscles and the corresponding movement of the dowsing instrument. Add to this the natural psychic, intuitive awareness that many people have developed, to one degree or another, of this life energy spectrum, so that they know the answer without recourse to dowsing, and one has a picture within the context of subtle energies and the subjective life we all lead.

Many dowsers know or can feel in their hand the condition of subtle health energies, for example. They do not need a pendulum except perhaps for verification. They just need to apply their mental concentration. The 'what should I do' kind of questions get answered, if they are not obscured by a pre-formed conscious or unconscious desire, by relating to the energy complex at the emotional/mental level which makes up our personality and knows the right answer for us. However, we usually have an answer in our minds, whenever we ask a question, and we only ask for verification. Hence, the pendulum can become inaccurate, because we are not able to accept an answer we do not want.

Another interesting phenomenon along these lines which firmly links dowsing to the unconscious, is knowing the time of day. Many people realize that one can programme one's mind to wake one up at a particular hour in the morning simply by impressing on one's mind to do so. Children often bang their heads on the pillow, say seven times, to wake up at seven o'clock. This is clearly using the unconscious to feed the conscious. Similarly, one can use a pendulum to dowse for the time of day if you do not have a watch, clearly tapping in to one's unconscious knowledge.

It is all a question of concentration. We do not, after all, remember all our knowledge and experiences *simultaneously*. This would drive us crazy! It is stored in our subconscious memory, ready for access upon demand. So, for knowledge which is more deeply buried, we need a prop or a ritual, an aide-memoire, to bring up the knowledge to consciousness. This explains too, how dowsers, often know the answer as soon as they bring out their pendulum or rods, but *before* they actually use them. The concentration or direction of mind, their intention, provides the conscious answer before the ritual of dowsing commences.

Actually, I do not really recommend the use of a pendulum for making personal decisions. Would it not be better to develop our own discrimination, intuition and higher mind rather than trying to abrogate the responsibility to a button on a string? David Tansley comments humourously, but with meaning, that emotional or indecisive people can get hooked (metaphorically) and definitely they should stop well before God starts giving instructions through their pendulum!

Dowsing Rates

Many aspects of dowsing require answers on a scale rather than or in addition to a simple 'yes' or 'no' response. When dowsing for water or mineral deposits, for example, the depth and physical characteristics, (quantity etc.) are also required. A qualitative feel for these factors may be determinable from the strength of the dowsing reaction, but exact details require a different approach. One can, using questions with a 'yes' or 'no' response, zero in on the required answer. Thus, for example, a water diviner having discovered an underground water source, will call out depths in feet, increasing first in five foot intervals until a positive reaction is discovered and then in one foot intervals to get the exact level.

This method is appropriate under such circumstances. However, when the 'choices' are multiple, as in medical dowsing or radiesthesia, a different approach is required. This may be both for the diagnosis of specific conditions as well as in the decision on which remedy to prescribe – as in homoeopathy, for example. Again, I believe one should seek a balance in the use of radiesthesia. We are not suggesting an abrogation of all the normal diagnostic and prescribing skills of the physician, but when honestly mystified or simply desiring corroboration, the use of a dowsing instrument can be of great value. It depends too on the therapist – some are far more gifted in this approach than others and can place more reliance upon it. Perhaps, too, the gap between the subconscious, the superconscious and the conscious mind in such people is considerably less than usual, intuition and direct psychic perception having a large part to play.

Radionics is the therapeutic science making the widest use of complex dowsing machines, described in the section below on sophisticated dowsing instruments. Here, a combination of dials, often 9, with each one having positions numbered from 0 to 9, is used, giving a series of possible rates from 000,000,000 to 999,999,999. The spatial arrangement of the dials is also considered of importance to the sensitivity and fine tuning of the instrument. The dials are turned until a positive dowsing response is achieved. By doing this in a logical fashion, it does not take long to find the correct settings. The meaning of these rates is determined for each machine, usually supplied within the operator's manual. For example, with the De La Warr radionic instrument, the rate for the stomach is 32, set in the first two dials, the second two dials represent the balance of function – 48 or 49 indicate normal function, while 46 or 47 would indicate underactivity. The rate for toxicity is 90222. Thus a reading of 32,46,90222 on the nine dials would represent an underactive stomach due to a toxic condition. The practitioner may not, of course, be starting from scratch with each patient. He would take a regular case history and use his other diagnostic skills to ascertain the problem.

The rate and cause of this toxic condition could then be further tested: 30337 in the last five digits, for example, indicates Botriocephalus, a species of tape worm.

Vernon Wethered in his book: *Medical Radiesthesia*, describes two other methods of determining rates for therapeutic purposes. Firstly, he uses a 100cm (one meter) ruler. The rule is placed on a table away from possible negative influences (electrical equipment etc.) and then supported on blocks. Wethered uses rubber blocks to 'insulate' the rule from stray influences. As we pointed out, dowsing is personal and whatever helps you has its validity and necessity for you in the search to tap the non-conscious information. Further blocks are placed alongside the rule so that remedy and patient samples can be placed upon them. A wooden meter rule can be obtained from most hardware shops and large neoprene 'corks' can be found in many chemists or wine-making shops. Wethered also places his samples in glass vials to act as 'resonators' and 'amplifiers'. Whether the vials amplify the vibration or psychologically help to tune and amplify the user's dowsing response (or a combination of both) is not so much of importance. The power of the user's concentrated mind would be enough to perform either or both of these functions.

A patient sample of saliva, blood spot or hair (this could be from yourself, in trials) is placed on a block at 0cms. Now move your pendulum along the rule until you get a positive response holding in mind that you are measuring your own level of vitality. 0cms means you should be dead, while 100cms means that you are in tip-top condition. Supposing the pendulum goes positive at 40cms and you feel you need a boost or a tonic. Holding each of the possible tonics in your left hand, in turn, now check your vitality rate once again. The tonic that gives you the highest reading will be the most valuable to you.

To discover the level of conditions other than vitality, a witness that relates to that condition is placed at the 100 cms mark and the balance point found. 100cms means that the condition is present in full and 0cms means that it is completely absent. 50cms makes a good average point to work to. In some circumstances, for example, the condition of the nervous system, one is looking for a reading of 50cms or more. To decide on a measure to boost the level, samples of possible remedies can be placed at the 0cms mark and readings taken until the remedy (or remedies) giving the maximum reading is found.

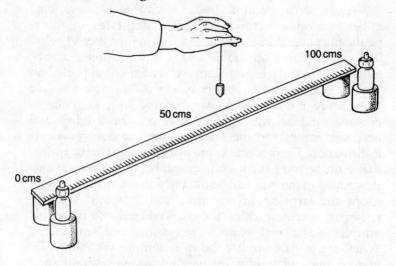

In the case of tests for toxic or diseased conditions, one is looking for a reading of 50cms or less and the best remedy will be the one that reduces the level of the condition to 50cms.

The choice of witnesses is dependant upon your own approach to dowsing. Wethered used quite a complex assortment of witnesses, acetyl choline (a naturally occurring compound in the nervous system) as a witness for testing the overall state of the nervous system, urea or uric acid for checking the general level of toxicity and so on. It depends upon what suits you and how intuitive or mental you are in your approach. It is quite possible, if you are sure of yourself, to simply use a piece of paper with the condition written down upon it as a witness, or just to hold the subject matter in mind while seeking your rate.

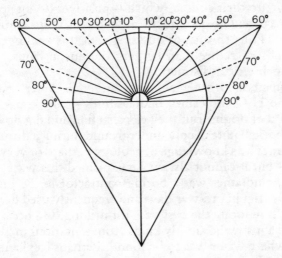

A similar system described fully in Vernon Wethered's book, employs a triangle, with the rate being determined from the angle along the inverted base relative to the central point within the triangle at which the pendulum is held. It is the direction of oscillation of the pendulum that determines the rate. Samples and witnesses can be placed at the three points of the triangle. Similar systems are used by Dr. Yao and others to determine vitamin and mineral deficiencies from a list of these supplements and a pie-chart representing the level of balance within the body and its requirements.

Animals, Dowsing and Subtle Energy Perception

So many of man's inventions and discoveries are later found to be already in biological use by other species that the possibility of 'dowsing' abilities in animals is not so silly. I do not of course, mean a polar bear with a dowsing rod looking for seals under the ice! Animals, as we know, do have senses that we do not. Fish, for example, which often orientate themselves upstream while hovering and looking for food, are not entirely dependant upon the flow of water for their sense of direction. Rivers usually have a weak electrical gradient running from the mouth, which is negative, to their source, which is positive. If you apply a similar current to an aquarium, the fish will swim 'upstream'. True, this is not dowsing, but it is energy detection, sensory rather than tapping the unconscious. Or is there such a clear distinction?

Elephants and other animals can smell water – detect airborne H_2O molecules one assumes – and know their direction of origin. But they can also find and dig down to water buried quite deeply underground during a drought – sometimes by a knowledge of geology perhaps or very faint smell – but it cannot always be explained this way.

My grandfather was a boring contractor in the English Lake District in pre-war days and frequently used diviners to help him locate the best sites for drilling. On occasions, he used a man who simply knew from sensations in his feet alone where water was to be found. Perhaps elephants can do the same, instinctively?

Plant roots, too, will seek out water and willow will even break into sealed drains. Every pet owner knows that dogs and cats, especially, have choices of where they like to sleep or lie, frequently based on no obvious visible reasons, while dowsers can often show that they are simply preferring places of positive or negative earth energies. Similarly, my wife and I are always amazed at the uncanny ability of mice to break into air-tight, sealed containers of their favourite goodies in our store cupboards, totally ignoring similar containers with less appetizing mouse food!

In this connection, it is worth mentioning the well-known T.C. Lethbridge, a Cambridge archaelogist, dowser and author, who developed a system of fixing rates for different substances using his pendulum in a novel manner, discovering some fascinating correlations amongst the lives of insects and animals. Lethbridge used a pendulum on a long string, up to 50 to 60 inches in length. First, he would roll up the thread onto a rod or pencil and then thinking of a substance, an object or an abstract idea (e.g. calcium, a cat or love) he would let the pendulum down from the rod, letting it swing backwards and forwards. At a certain length, the pendulum would hesitate and within half an inch it would start to move in a circle. Lethbridge measured the length of the string at this point and also counted how many gyrations the pendulum made before returning to its forwards and backwards motion. Thus each thing tested had two co-ordinates, or *rates*, expressed as, for example, the colour grey at 22:7 – twenty-two inches and seven gyrations, while silver was 22:22. This system clearly gives one a multiple answer situation from a pendulum, an improvement on a simple 'yes' or 'no', when detailed analysis is required. Whether there is anything absolute about the numbers or whether any arbitary scale would suffice, I do not know. Numerologists might have some answers here, but Lethbridge thought that it might be absolute. Certainly, it was reproducible for himself and others who adopted the system.

Lethbridge took the rates of many, many things, discovering as he did so some fascinating correlations. You may have noticed for example that silver is grey, and they both have the primary rate of 22, and so does lead. Sometimes, however, materials and ideas were on the same rate, but without any apparent correlation at all. His system worked in practice too. He could take any arbitrary piece of turf and, using his pointing finger as an antenna or 'radar' aerial, he could accurately determine, by a series of pendulum rate tests what was out of sight, under the turf.

Thus heartened by his new and versatile system, Lethbridge discovered that, for example, an insect would have the same rates as its food plant. We are now coming onto the familiar territory of vibratory resonance. Dr. Lethbridge's findings give us a clue as to how animals (and humans!) know things *instinctively*. Is *instinct* partially a function of *awareness of vibration?* How for example, does a rare insect find its way to a rare food plant? What is the mechanism that draws it? What is its unconscious radar beacon? We are also back with the moths that zero in on a female from 30 miles away when the pheromone concentration is down to one molecule. Do these 'senses' actually respond to the specific vibration of molecules rather than chemical reactions? This would certainly explain how such an infinitesimal concentration can be detected, if the detection is an *informational trigger* to seeking the female, rather than being required to enter into a more biochemical process.

Lethbridge's discoveries surpassed themselves with his analysis of cats' whiskers. Let us quote in his own words, from his last book, published posthumously, *The Power of the Pendulum*:

'We have a Siamese cat and this almost completely wild animal is a great hunter. On most mornings before we get up she comes into the bedroom and goes to sleep on the end of the bed. One morning she sat up with a jerk and began to scan the corner of the room. She seemed to fix a bearing, jumped off the bed and ran out of the open door. In about three minutes she was back with a short-tailed field vole, which she devoured with horrid noises under the bed.

'Now, on her line of bearing, there is a grassy bank beside the lane, about twenty-five yards from where she was sleeping. To get there, she had to run along a passage in the opposite direction, across a big bedroom, down the back-stairs, across the kitchen, out of the window, through a small court, round two sides of the house and then across a yard. It seemed clear that she had picked up the position of the vole in her sleep and then fixed this on her waking mind. At least two mental levels were involved. She kept that bearing in her mind through several changes in direction and knew exactly where the vole was. It had no chance of escape. This has happened several times since then, and the same revolting ritual feast has taken place beneath our bed.

'It seemed probable that the cat's whiskers acted like divining rods and I decided to try and find out their co-ordinates in our pendulum code. There is more work in this than anyone might think, for not only have you to rate the whiskers but you have to find out to what thought forms these co-ordinates also belong. Actually the cat has at least four sets of bristles. The longest and furthest back have a rate of 16 inches for sex, which is not a surprise. The next group is on 20 inches. Man comes on this rate, with love and life. The smallest and farthest forward of the groups is on 24 inches. On this rate you also find mice. Finally, its eyebrows are on 10 inches. On 10 inches you find heat, explaining surely how a cat knows with unerring certainty where to find the warmest spot in the house.

'The four groups of bristles, then, seem to explain a cat's vigorous sex life; its fondness for mankind; its passion for mice and its love of warmth (Figure 4). This can hardly be

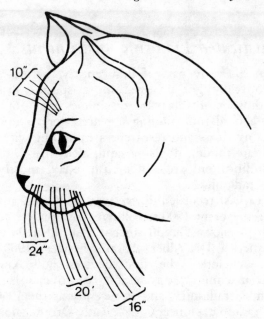

Figure 4. Diagram of a cat's face to show the rates of its whiskers as indicated by the pendulum: 10" = heat and light; 16" = sex; 20" = living things and man; 24" = small mammals.

'either chance or coincidence, but looks like a carefully planned arrangement. If you were asked to describe the characteristics of a cat, surely these four would come high on your list.'

And one further piece of the jigsaw puzzle. A cat's whiskers are made of keratin, which we know has piezo-electric properties, connected in pigeons and other animals with the bio-electronic energy system. Add to this the fact that the length of an aerial (or antenna if you are American) reflects its resonance or transmission/receiving wavelengths. Nothing is ever haphazard in Nature. There must be a purpose for the number and lengths of cat's whiskers. Perhaps Samson had a point when he refused to have his hair cut – or is that simply being too bizarre?

So, there we have it, dowsing is yet another aspect of vibrational resonance and tuning. It all fits so beautifully together. I just cannot believe that a cat's whiskers, of which it takes such great care, are purely for vanity and for measuring the spaces between cupboards!

Sophisticated Dowsing Instruments

Back in the early part of this century, before scientific research really got grooved in to specific disciplines, (with those more abstruse disciplines that got left out having a hard time finding a place later), a number of private inventors and researchers came out with sophisticated rate-finding dowsing equipment that with only a few modifications are still in use today, mostly in the field of radionics.

The earliest recorded device was the American Osciloclast of the early 1900's, followed by devices from the English physician Guyon Richards, in the 1920's.

In America, Dr. Albert Abrams between 1900 and the 1920's, developed the first devices now known as radionic machines. Considerable controversy has always surrounded radionics, and as recently as the 1960's, one of the radionic pioneers, Dr. Ruth Drown along with her staff were sent to jail after a court case brought by the American Food and Drug Administration. I wonder if there is a case for sending the manufacturers of drugs with harmful and undiscovered side effects to jail? One thinks of DDT, opren, thalidomide, contraceptive pills and *hundreds more, if not thousands*. That might make them think twice! Or will they say that *full* and *thorough* testing is impossible because of all the ramifications and possibilities? But then why throw good people, like Dr Drown and her colleagues, into jail – who no doubt had many satisfied clients and patients? Even that beautiful and wonderful herbalist, Dr. Christopher did time in jail, though he did use the time for writing down some of his precious accumulated wisdom into his classic books on herbalism.

Strangely enough, in 1949, Thomas G. Hieronymus received his patent, number 2,482,773, for the *Detection of Emanations from Materials, and Measurements of the Volumes Thereof*, the first patent ever issued for such a device and although the laws of conventional physics cannot explain how these devices work!

The basic design behind such instruments is as follows:

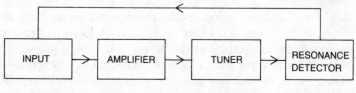

The circuit consists of an *input* device on which the sample under test is positioned, this could be a simple flat plate or coil covered with plastic. Then an ordinary *amplifier*, followed by a *tuning* phase, normally consisting of a number of potentiometers. The relative positions of these potentiometers gives one a number or the *rate* for the sample. Nine potentiometers with readings from 0 to 9, for example, would give numbers in the range 000,000,000 to 999,999,999. Then there is the *resonance detector* with which the user interfaces. Usually this consists of a flat sheet of bakelite, plexiglass or other material under which is placed a spirally wound coil, connected back into the input coil or plate. Based on a tactile response in the finger when rubbed on the detector, tuning is achieved when the finger *sticks*. This corresponds to a resonant link between the sample, the tuning phase and the detection plate with the user's own unconscious mind or energies. Sometimes the detector is once again a pendulum oscillating over the detector plate, which reads positive when the correct setting is located for each potentiometer.

Most of these radionics machines are decidedly pre-war in design, built like an old-fashioned radio and there is scope for a neat and modern digital radionics dowsing instrument, a project that I am currently researching, and where an understanding of modern scalar wave theory (see chapter 11) should prove of value.

Subtle Energy Photography.

The desire to capture on permanent, visible record the subtle emanations from the body is understandable and no doubt would have value, in the same way that an EEG or ECG of the brain and heart gives us an indication of how these organs are getting along. Let us not forget, however, that we are dealing with a fluid, flexible and highly tenuous energy system and any attempt to crystallize our knowledge of it may fix our beautiful butterfly into a grim death-mask of its living vibrancy. What is needed are sensitive physicians who can see and use these things, not so much sensitive photographic emulsions – though these too would no doubt have their uses.

Kirlian photography is certainly the most well publicized of these techniques. But before one gets carried away, the question must be sincerely asked as to *what* is being photographed. Energy has its own level and it does not readily seem possible that finer emotional, mental or higher auric emanations can be captured at a physical level. At the most, we are working at the dividing line between the bio-electronic energy system and the etheric level, which will, of course, reflect the higher energies to some degree.

As Kirlian photography is currently practised in most Western systems, it has another serious problem. Emanations from fingers and leaves are photographed by placing a dielectric plate on top of an electrode. The film is located on top of this, emulsion side uppermost and the hand, finger, leaf or other subject is placed on top. *A very high voltage* at low current is then applied to the electrode and through the plate. The resulting photographs, which can be spectacular and beautiful, are therefore a result of the *interactions* between the subject and a high voltage. One of the main problems with all sensitive scientific measurement is that the *process of measurement changes what is being measured*. And I cannot believe that the very small electrical fields around the body and its other electrical and magnetic characteristics are not changed by the application of a high voltage.

Secondly, there is a perfectly understandable and rational physical explanation of the so-called Kirlian results, as a corona discharge – the excitation of electrons leading on their return to a lower energy to an emission of light, as well as secondary radiation such as X-rays. It is these emissions that cause most of the patterns on this kind of 'Kirlian' photograph.

However, the case is not at all closed. According to Scott Hill, who visited the Soviet Union in 1976, co-authoring the book *The Cycles of Heaven*, the real Kirlian equipment was and is far more sophisticated. Their equipment has the following noise-reducing factors:

1. The film is *at a distance* from the electrodes and the soup of excited electrons.

2. The light from the discharge is enlarged, filtered, focused and analyzed *before* reaching the film. It represents about 15% of the original light.

3. The biological object is itself made of one of the electrodes.

4. The whole equipment is done in an atmosphere of known composition, thus eliminating unknown spectral emissions from excited gas molecules. Moreover, great care is taken to exclude experimental variables such as skin moisture, variations in electrode pressure and so on.

The Russians are well aware of the defects even of this equipment, 'But,' says, Dr. Inyushin, 'it is one of the few means available for diagnosing the bio-plasma. With the aid of the Kirlian effect, it has been possible to penetrate into a new field of knowledge, using the latest achievements of quantum electronics to obtain unique information about the bioenergetic state of the organism, and to prove the existence of the biofield'. (From *Biostimulation Through Laser Radiation and Bioplasma* by V.M. Inyushin and P.R. Chekurov, published by the Danish Society for Psychical Research, 1977, Copenhagen, translated by Scott Hill & T.D. Ghoshal).

So while it might be fun to have a western-style Kirlian photograph taken and analyzed, one should not take too seriously the 'diagnosis' given. The practitioners themselves are normally aware that even two photographs taken within minutes of each other are often quite radically different, depending upon skin conductivity and moisture, body electrical charge and other environmental factors. One can understand how these beautiful patterns can be taken as meaningful, but their real nature must be understood. A friend of mine was told at an analysis of a Kirlian photograph taken at an exhibition, that she was not using her spiritual potential due to the negative effect of her family. As a result she got angry with her husband and children and nearly left them. I wonder if folk realize the effect of such irresponsible 'diagnoses' on their clients?

Vibrational Science & Harnessing Subtle Energies

Harnessing Subtle Energies

It has been a dream of mine for many years to figure out some way of transforming the energy within matter into useful power for heating, lighting, locomotion and all other power needs. I touched on this topic rather lightly in the chapter on crystals, resonance and modern physics but although one comes across stories from time to time of people who are supposed to have done this, there is never anything concrete to follow up.

Modern nuclear power stations convert a tiny amount of matter into usable energy, transforming it to electrical energy for relay around the country. Think how much better it would be if this could be done within one's own home by some safe means. To be frank, every home already has such a wonderful instrument, that can convert matter into heat and motive power. It is called a human being! And most of us are somewhat safer and produce less toxic waste than a nuclear power plant. The problem is: how to externalize this force of energy transformation into a device that needs no human energy to drive it.

There are those who can of their own concentration perform conscious miracles. This is normally a waste of spiritual power, but it is quite possible. When the mind becomes concentrated and gains conscious control of any of the inner centres, then all the energies below that level come into conscious possession and can be manipulated at will.

There are those too, who perform unconscious miracles. That is, their subtle constitution is such that the force of their own desire and will-power unconsciously harnesses these energies and makes things happen. This, perhaps, is one of the causes of 'poltergeists', often associated with the emotional life of a young adolescent. John Keely, born in 1837 and dying in 1898, was a man who strove all his life to harness the subtle energies into a motive force that would work consistently and independently of himself. That Keely could transmute subtle energies was without a doubt. He was able to provide convincing enough demonstrations to businessmen to raise five million dollars over five years to back his research – imagine how much that was worth, over a century ago. He flew a model zeppelin weighing eight pounds around the room using the transformed power from a note played on a violin. Using the same source, he could also start and run a twenty-five horse power motor. Using what he called this vibro-molecular or vibro-atomic force, he could float a solid iron ball on water and turn a seventy-two pound pulley. He also practically killed himself and blew his laboratory to pieces on more than one occasion. But he never managed to make any of these devices work without himself being present.

Ultimately, his backers became impatient and demanded, by court order, a full written record of his work for others to complete. This he refused to do and finally he was jailed for contempt of court.

The only other recorded history of someone harnessing subtle energies for physical power is Wilhelm Reich. Born is Austria in 1897, Reich initially studied psychology and psychiatry. A man of outspoken and often deviant views, both professional and political, Reich found it more comfortable to move to America, which he did in the 1930's.

During his time as a psychiatrist, Reich's own psychic abilities developed and he became able to see some of the auric energies and subtle energy emanations. This energy he called Orgone energy, describing it in much the same way as both ancient and modern yogis, sages and clairvoyants.

Both Reich and Keely had one basic theory in common, that of atmospheric subtle energies in the form of corpuscles. Keely developed this into a complex theory giving many names to it, including the vibro-molecular, vibro-atomic and dynaspheric force. Reich used the word bions, also known as vitality globules. On some days, especially by the sea-side, in the mountains or in the desert, you can actually see these globules of light dancing like small worms in a mosquito-esque manner and disappearing after just a few seconds. You might think they are spots before your eyes, but they are not always there and you cannot see them if you go indoors. But go outside and there they are again.

Vitality globules are said to be due to an infusion of the chemical oxygen with prana or life-force, from within, giving them an intense white light. One form of this prana, of which there are a number of varieties or vibrations, is associated with subtle energies originating in the sun. This solar prana supplies life forms with energy nourishment, partially through direct assimilation into our biophysical energy system and partially through the energizing and creation of these vitality globules – which are thus more visible on sunny days. This, perhaps, is another reason why during a dull winter and long periods of rain and cloud, we develop a tendency towards low energy in our mind-emotion-body complex, because the atmospheric concentration of solar prana falls when the sun cannot shine. It is also a fact that the spleen has an important subtle counterpart or sub-chakra with considerable responsibility for the bodily assimilation and distribution of environmental subtle energy, including these vitality globules.

Actually, it is unclear from his writings, whether Reich was referring to these airborne vitality globules or to a more universal infusion of gross matter with subtle. Reich did, however, discover that by making a box out of alternate layers of organic and inorganic material, he could trap this orgone energy inside, much like the heating effect in a greenhouse, where the heat can get in, but not out. This he called an orgone accumulator, which he used for his research. A modification of this device, he called a *shooter,* which was really a tube to direct the orgone energy from an accumulator to specific parts of the body for therapeutic purposes, with some considerable success.

Theorizing that the negative effects of radioactivity could be due to disruptions and disharmonies in the orgone or subtle energies, Reich thought that if he put a radioactive sample into an orgone accumulator the positive, health-giving orgone would counterbalance the negative nature of radioactivity. The full and horrifying, yet fascinating story is written up in Reich's Orgone Bulletin covering the period, summarized in Aubrey Westlake's book: *Pattern of Health.*

Reich and his researchers first put their radioactive sample inside a one-fold orgone charger. This was placed inside a twenty-layered orgone accumulator inside the orgone laboratory, itself lined with orgone amplifying materials. At that time, the background level of radioactivity was not measured, there being no reason for them to have predicted what was about to occur. Within a few hours however, the level of background radioactivity around the accumulator had risen alarmingly high. For some days, they continued the experiment, until Reich and his staff realised that they were getting ill, with symptoms of nausea, dizziness and headaches, while the air in the laboratory at times turned bluish. In fact, one of Reich's staff members nearly died after putting her head inside the accumulator for cleaning purposes.

But more bad news was to come. Firstly, they had a mass death of laboratory mice and then they discovered that the increased background level of radioactivity had spread over a distance of 500 square miles. The equipment was immediately dismantled and slowly Reich and his team returned, not only to full health, but to a level of increased health and well-being new to them all.

Reich's understanding of what had occurred was that the normally positive or friendly orgone energy (OR) became negative and destructive, Deadly Orgone energy (DOR), under the influence of the powerful negative radiations of the radioactive material. Their return to a state of powerful well-being and health, he attributed to the positive orgone energy 'fighting back' against the negative or deadly orgone energy, at least within their own bodies. One wonders what the results of Reich's experiments would have been had he had access to Dr. Yao's Pulsors and been able to reverse the subtle energy polarities and disharmonies. Unfortunately, the follow-up and more controlled experimentation that was so clearly indicated was never carried out, for the controversy that Reich provoked due to his work and scathing writings, eventually led to his downfall. He was summoned to court on a trivial charge, but failed to turn up, since he felt that an uninformed judiciary were in no position to pass judgement on advanced scientific experimentation. After further summonses and fines, he was eventually jailed for two years for contempt of court.

Reich's laboratories were destroyed, his writings burnt and banned from publication. Fortunately, some of his writings, already in the hands of interested people, have survived including the newsletters sent out concerning his research.

Reich did not believe that the authorities would let him live and indeed he died in jail, reputed to be of natural causes. Amongst Reich's other work was his 'cloudbuster' with which he was able to cause the rain to fall in the Arizona desert after setting up his equipment near a water source. Also, like Keely, he claimed to have developed a means of harnessing the 'motor power'! How this was done was never committed to paper, perhaps wisely, so we will never know how or if he really did it.

Reich was a true, natural researcher, but one cannot help but feel that he had strong negative and self-destructive forces in him. No situation or experiment is totally devoid of the personal factor and the more subtle the experiment, the more powerful these factors can become. How much of the energy he experimented with came from himself and his fellow sensitives, and how much from the 'bions' is impossible to know now.

I feel convinced that these subtle forces can be harnessed for mankind's benefit, but perhaps it will only come to pass when as dwellers on this planet we have the ability to handle such power for our own good. Resistance to change, greed, prejudice, sheer violence and desire for power, irrational political idealism – all these things mean that human beings are not yet ready to handle such tremendous power. But one day, perhaps, we human children will grow into a more loving and caring harmony with the great forces of Nature. I can see no other way except disaster out of our current world dilemma.

A Six Dimensional Universe

However, before technology can really approach and develop new methodologies in the subtle realms, there must first exist a theoretical and probably mathematical model upon which to develop such ideas. And the more a model or theory relates to the inner reality of the cosmos, the truer and more powerful it will be.

It must therefore include the vertical, creative energy spectrum in its thinking and I take the liberty of suggesting one such model here, based upon dimensionality.

Extra dimensions to our outer reality are concepts with which science fiction writers and mathematicians have long experimented, to such a degree that we forget the basics of what a 'dimension' actually is. I would define a dimension as an aspect in which 'reality' as we experience it and conceptualize about it, manifests itself. It is essentially employable as a mathematical or logical concept and each dimension identified allows us to specifically and mathematically define the 'dimensionality' of an object – its 'place' or manifestation within the dimensions chosen.

Thus, every object has a position in 'space' defined by three dimensions of distance all at right angles to each other. Between them, these three dimensions allow us to define, exactly, *where* something is and how *big* it is. These three dimensions are *lateral* (side to side), *vertical* (up and down) and *forwards/backwards*.

Mathematicians define them as the x, y and z axes of movement and location, thus:

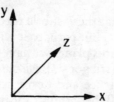

In addition to this, our physical universe changes with *time*. In fact, movement and difference automatically exist in time. Time is an essential aspect of duality, of polarity, of the observer and the observed being separate. This is why in the total Oneness of the Source, we say that it is the Eternal Now, there is no change. So time is a fourth dimension which we use to define 'reality.'

Now we have pointed out many times that 'nothing' comes from 'nothing' – you cannot get 'something' for 'nothing', that outward, physical reality is substantiated from within through a vertical energy spectrum leading back to the source, the eternal changelessness, the Creator within all manifest existence, the God within every particle and vibration of the Universe, within and without. So the energy patterns within, affect – indeed create – the outward manifestation.

Similarly, we have also observed that what is without affects the patterns within.

This does, therefore, give us essentially two further dimensions in our view of any event or object – the direction of creation from the within to the without and the completion of the energy circuit, from the without to the within, both dimensions being along the vertical, creative, energy spectrum or direction. These may be called, quite simply, the *inward* and *outward* dimensions.

So every event is positioned in three-dimensional space, it is constantly changing in time, it is substantiated or takes its existence from within and it affects the inner energies whenever its outward four dimensions are altered. We have therefore a six dimensional universe.

Now, all of this would be only of theoretical interest and of little practical use if it did not also provide a means of understanding physical events in a deeper fashion, as well as, ultimately, opening up a way of working with matter for the creation of new instrumentation and devices that can provide us with an energy source or improve our health and well-being. I'm not a mathematician or a physicist, but the concept, since it relates correctly to 'reality', must surely have some scientific power and relevance?

As I write, we are watching the aftermath of the Russian Chernobyl nuclear disaster. It is very clear that we have to find safer ways of transforming the energy inherent in matter. We need greater subtlety in our approach. And until scientific thinking understands the essential *simplicity* inherent in natural processes – its simple polarity and movement and creation from within – we will always be struggling under the feeling that to get a lot you have to do a lot, a reflection of the old and incorrect adage, that hard work leads to riches. It is simply not true. All that is required is the right action at the right time, in the right place. One would like to know, scientifically speaking, just what that right action, place and timing were!

Relativity, Quantum Mechanics and an Ordered Universe

Albert Einstein, formulator of a deterministic, mathematical and general scientific/philosophical understanding of the laws underlying space, time and energy, expressed his appreciation of the probabalistic nature of the apparently opposing, yet equally powerful concepts of quantum mechanics in his oft-quoted remark, 'I cannot beleive that God plays dice with the Universe'. Much of the endeavour of modern theoretical physicists is to unify these two apparently conceptually opposite theories, both of which remain extant because each has a powerful ability to describe and predict energetic events in the physical universe.

But let us look a little closer at determinism and probability. We toss a coin and say that it is chance whether it lands heads or tails. What we mean is that *within the confines of only heads or tails*, we can expect a random distribution. But how random is random when there are only two choices? In other words, the probabalistic aspect of the event is underlain by a deterministic order.

Similarly, in all aspects of probability and statistical analysis, the appreciation of *patterns* is fundamental. Stockbrokers and insurance companies as well as all kinds of lottery are run with a full knowledge of the patterns that are likely to develop. This appreciation that there are patterns underlying so-called random events means that there exists an underlying principle or law – something deterministic, a part of the manifestation of karma, cause and effect – *something that is not random*. The use of 'laws' of probability inherently require a deterministic substrate or order. Whether – or to what depth – we understand that law is another matter.

Similarly, the mathematical formulations of quantum mechanics are a powerful means of describing events at a physical level, just as the formulations of statistical probability are an excellent way of describing the fall of a dice or a coin. But underlying it is a field of energy, structured through unknown forces following the universal principles of polarity and cause and effect – the basic laws of energy interactions. It is an approach to those as yet undescribed forces that will bring about a fusion of relativity theory and quantum mechanics. So I would say that Einstein was right, God does not play dice with the universe, He just appears to do so from our restricted point of view.

Actually, the whole concept which believes in the randomness of the cosmos seems to be lacking in basic observation of nature. Do we not see a wonderful panorama of order, structure and patterning from the behaviour of sub-atomic matter, to crystals, to biochemistry, to the intricacies of life-forms, to planets, stars and galaxies? If probability reigned supreme then there would have to be an infinite number of possibilities of everything for the theory to hold good. Such a concept appears ludicrous and is certainly not the state of affairs as we find them. Probability theory requires order and determinism for it to have any meaning. It is like a theory that describes the behaviour of bubbles on the surface of water and is so focused on them that it fails to notice the great ocean giving them existence. But this is the way with all great scientific milestones – it is only obvious when pointed out to us!

Scalar Electromagnetic Theory and Virtual Field Engineering

In yogic, mystical perception and understanding, both the physical, observable, universe as well as the higher or inner regions are said to be manifested out of *Prakriti*. Prakriti is primal energy or nature, the prime cause or essence of material substance. Matter, in the outwardly, scientific sense, is its final outward expression. Prakriti is that which gives form to the creative power of the One, known as Shabd, when it reaches the realm of Universal Mind. Form is, in a sense, the result of stress and strain, manifesting within the primal prakriti, under the influence of the three gunas or modes of duality. Prakriti is, so to speak, the first form that manifests within the higher materio-mental region. All other forms are derived from it.

This understanding of Primal Energy and the formation of 'lower' vibrations and form due to stress, or locked-in potential, within the more subtle realm or dimension, is at the basis of probably the most exciting scientific theory of matter, energy and material phenomena yet formulated. It is called the *Scalar Electromagnetic Theory*.

One of its major protagonists and developers is Lt. Colonel Thomas Bearden – a theoretical physicist, and nuclear engineer, now retired from military service but who has spent much of his life working in American defence circles. About half of Dr. George Yao's book, *Pulsor – Miracle of Microcrystals* consists of a fascinating non-mathematical exposition of this Scalar Electromagnetic Theory, written by Bearden.

Supporters of conventional modern physics, relativity and quantum mechanics suffer from an essential flaw in understanding when they think that there exists a *fundamental* field of existence within the confines of material observation – when they say that matter and force do indeed come out of nowhere and that nothing exists beyond that. Mathematical and philosophical concepts are familiar with the attempt to demonstrate that 'coming out of nowhere' is understandable, but as yet theoretical physicists and mathematicians have been unable to provide satisfactory and unified laws of material existence based on this premise. And not surprisingly.

Scalar electromagnetics (EM) on the other hand, has clearly arisen from scientists who are aware of deeper and inner dimensions to their own life, whose consciousness and experience has embraced higher experience and who are therefore aware that most theories in modern physics are fundamentally lacking in an appreciation that energies are created from within, and exist within.

Scalar EM theory does not supplant Einsteinian relativity and quantum mechanics, but it does show it to be a special case, able to describe certain material phenomena, but incomplete, much in the same way that Einstein did not make Newton's understanding obsolete or incorrect, but simply placed it in a wider context.

Scalar EM research is continuing and is capable of scientific verification through the creation of advanced devices and instrumentation that can be seen to work. Bearden claims that the Russians have been working on scalar electromagnetic instrumentation for many years and already possess a considerably armoury of such energy devices. This new research seems to me to be the most far-reaching advance in scientific understanding since the formulation of relativity during the early years of this century (1905–1915) and quantum mechanics in 1926.

One of its primary concepts is that any apparent zero or 'no-thing' (such as vacuum), can be constituted of an infinite number of *substructures* which all sum to zero, giving the *appearance* of 'no-thing' while actually consisting of 'some-thing' real. Conventional theory regards the point at which forces sum to zero *as* zero, while scalar EM is able to understand each zero as substructurally different.

Thus:

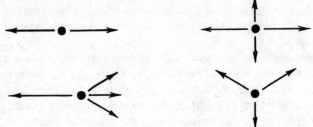

are all the same at the zero point, but are all quite different in substructure.

Two or more electric or magnetic fields, for example, may sum to zero, but the zero point, though absent of field effects, contains a stressed, or locked-in potential that reflects the summation of the substructure. Any 'unbalanced' variations in the constitution of this substructure will result in observable field effects and whilst conventional physics expresses this as the field itself, the new approach recognizes the importance of the potentials that have created the field. Potentials are thus regarded as 'real things', while fields are simply effects. This is a reversal of the conventional approach, where potential is generally described in terms of its effect and is not regarded as the 'real thing'.

In more specific terms, what we may think of as 'empty' vacuum is actually 'packed full' of potential, summed to zero, in a stable state, giving us the illusion of there being 'nothing there'. This is known as the *virtual* state of *electrostatic scalar potential*, a scalar value being one characterized by magnitude only, i.e. potential without manifestation. In fact, while virtual states are a familiar concept to modern physics, the new theory takes the idea considerably further.

As we have previously described, modern physics is already aware that matter as we perceive it is mostly 'vacuum' or 'space', and whilst this space is conventionally seen to contain sub-atomic particles and fields, scalar EM and other theories that conceptualize a virtual state, perceive that these particles and fields are actually due to activities in the virtual or scalar substructure.

This physically unobservable energy, Bearden has called *anenergy. And it is changes within the substructure of the stressed, locked-in, potential of the virtual state or anenergy that give rise to observable phenomena, to our outwardly perceptible physical universe.*

Furthermore, vacuum is, in the new theory, equatable with the relativistic concept of *spacetime*, the curvature of which in conventional relativity, due to the presence of mass, results in gravitational effects. Bearden's anenergy can therefore be thought of as *spatio-temporal stress*.

Indeed, Bearden explains how mass, charge, spin, sub-atomic particles, electric fields, magnetic fields, the speed of light, gravitation and all the basic forces and phenomena of our physical world are directly related to and arise from variations and patternings in the virtual state.

Furthermore, the virtual state does itself manifest from higher or more inwardly nested virtual states, reaching up to the levels of mental energy.

The virtual state of electrostatic scalar potential is thus the subtle energy blueprint, which we have been discussing at length in this book and this new approach provides us with a scientific basis for understanding all subtle physical phenomena.

The atmosphere of a place, for example, is a subtle encoding of the virtual energy patterns which still sum together in the same way, producing the same outwardly observable phenomena, whilst being different in their inner or infolded substructure.

Since, at a still higher level, the virtual state includes mental energies, this provides an explanation of how the vibrational encoding of any place or object can contain a pattern of the individuals who have used it, together with their emotions and motivations, i.e. an understanding of psychometry, the ability to read vibrations. It also gives a basis to my 'sub-atomic fingerprint' idea described in chapter six. It shows too, how food takes on a character from those who cook it, since the mental intentions, motives, mood and character will all become encoded into the subtle or virtual substructure of the food itself, affecting those who eat it, entraining their energies in a similar manner through resonance. It is often said that the one who cooks in a house, holds the key to the harmony of the people living there and that food prepared in a mood of concentration and spiritual love will enhance the consciousness of all those who eat it. This indeed is the more inward meaning of 'blessing', or saying grace – the inner change beyond the ritual – that can induce an uplifting effect.

But scalar electromagnetic theory does more than provide an understanding of mechanisms by which manifestation can take place, for, being a true scientific theory, it contains the mathematics and physics required to *engineer the virtual state*, in order to create effects at the gross physical or observable level. Using relativistic concepts, but seen in the light of the new approach, it describes how, by summing electric and magnetic fields to zero, the conservation of energy principle results in a 'bleed off' into certain aspects of the gravitational field, through the medium of the virtual condition. In other words, by manipulating the electromagnetic effects of the virtual substructure, this substructure can itself be *deterministically* and *quantifiably* altered, resulting in changes in the observable, physical 'reality'.

Such scalar electromagnetic engineering is already the subject of experimentation and provides too, a theoretical basis for genuine 'free-energy' machines. The concept of 'free-energy' machines has conventionally been laughed off the stage because they apparently violate the laws of energy conservation by assuming that one can get something for nothing. This is, of course, correct, but the new approach allows one to both perceive and mathematically formulate that if the locked-in potential of the virtual or subtle state can be engineered into manifestation, then the apparent gain in energy at the observable level is counterbalanced by the release of stress or loss of potential in the virtual. The laws of energy conservation are thus satisfied.

Note that such virtual substructure engineering

theoretically permits both materialization and dematerialization of not only electromagnetic phenomena, but also of mass, charge, spin etc., i.e. 'objects'. For mass itself is conceived of as a standing *scalar wave* in the virtual state, trapped by particle spin. The scalar wave or pattern in the virtual condition, being set up by internal resonance within the mass. It is therefore theoretically possible to dematerialize objects and rematerialize them elsewhere by engineering their physical existence into the virtual state and then 'releasing the tension', permit re-materialization at another location, by simply modulating the spatial parameters of material existence. Bearden mentions a number of his colleagues who have preliminary 'free-energy' devices working, have achieved scalar transmutation of chemical elements, have lifted heavy weights by antigravity and so on. One is reminded of both Keely and Reich, both of whom had clearly stumbled onto scalar wave engineering without fully understanding its implications.

Scalar waves, longitudinal pressure waves in the potential energy of the virtual state, may be generated by a number of methods including both electromagnetic and mechanical stress. When two such scalar waves are deterministically created and beamed such that, like two searchlights, they overlap at a distance from their source, then the interaction or interference of these two virtual waves can produce observable energy at that point by a process Bearden calls by the imaginatively expressive word 'kindling'. Anenergy is 'kindled' into observable energy – electromagnetic, sub-atomic particles, mass and so on. This technique is known as *scalar wave interferometry*, and again, the Russians are said to be experts in this technology.

Systems which can transform electromagnetic energy into subtle energy or scalar waves and vice versa, Bearden calls *translators* and they include, he says, plasmas, ionized gases, stressed crystals, Pulsors®, Reich's orgone boxes, scalar interferometers, some semi-conductive materials, dielectric capacitors and so on.

The earth itself, he suggests, is a giant scalar wave generator with multiple resonances, and earth energies are therefore subtle scalar waves associated with both mineral content and physical stress. Indeed, many UFO

(Unidentified Flying Objects), ball lightning and other phenomena can be explained as random scalar wave interference from earth-stress generated scalar waves which, meeting in the atmosphere kindle the formation of electromagnetic energy in the visible spectrum. This hypothesis is given further weight by the fact that these kind of phenomena are often associated with particular geological areas, especially granite, which has both a crystalline structure and a higher than average radioactive content. Sudden bursts of 'UFO' activity may thus be a kind of scalar wave earthquake or stress-related phenomenon.

UFO's are often said to respond to human intelligence, moving according to the thoughts of the observer and even this becomes understandable because thought or mind energy are a higher vibration of scalar waves and are harmonically tunable to observed phenomena. The kindling, subtle energy producing the 'UFO' could thus become readily latched into the thoughts of the observer, moving and manifesting accordingly.

In fact, Bearden suggests that the two halves of the human cerebrum act as scalar wave generators and detectors, with electrical brain waves being just the 'residue' of scalar wave activity. He points out, too, that all activity in the nervous system is essentially scalar in origin and that the neuronal synaptic system is ideal for scalar wave generation while if nature had really intended the nervous-system to be primarily a conductor of electricity, we would have been endowed with straight wire conductors or their equivalent.

This understanding underlies the psychotronic devices said to be used by the Soviet Union for the manipulation of world mood. The 'woodpecker' signal previously discussed, for example, actually being scalar in its active, virtual nature and possessing harmonics that relate to levels of mental or emotional scalar anenergy. Similarly, the vibrational patterns of disease are encoded at a scalar level and can theoretically be broadcast.

In this respect, too, the poltergeist activity mentioned earlier in this chapter as seemingly associated with the emotional life of children and adolescents can be understood as the subconscious projection of scalar wave activity, resulting in the spontaneous movement of objects. Similarly, the ectoplasm and materialization of spiritualists and mediums that can accompany the communication by the medium with whatever or whoever they are in contact.

Vitality globules, too, are most likely due to a kindling of subtle energy, producing light as a bi-product, or maybe these bright and evanescent sparks are points of interference in a grid pattern of multiple scalar waves permeating the atmosphere at that time. I have myself noticed that their appearance is often linked to the build up of electrical tension before summer storms, when they become particularly numerous.

Some cosmic, sub-atomic particles, too, may owe part of their origin to spontaneous kindling out of the energy-rich, potential of vacuum in outer space.

In fact, an understanding of how phenomena can materialize, how material substance reflects its internal virtual, scalar or subtle substructure and how electromagnetic forces are like bubbles or waves forming on the surface of the virtual energy ocean, permits understanding in a scientific mode of many previously inexplicable phenomena.

Lethbridge's cat's whiskers with piezo-electric properties are seen to have scalar wave detection capabilities, in the new terminology. The same will be true of the 'sixth sense' and indeed all vibrational awareness found in both humans and lower species. Since scalar waves pass through all substances at the gross physical level, sensory apparatus on the exterior of the body is not necessarily required and one imagines that the brain and central nervous system themselves are tuned for scalar wave detection.

Ball lightning (see pages 92–93) could also be a kindling phenomenon from virtual anenergy, created out of a vortex which for some reason forms a temporarily self-sustaining complex from which electromagnetic energy manifests at visible wavelengths. One wonders how long it will be before there is a generation of childrens' toys making use of kindling technology to produce a wide variety of kaleidoscopic and other patternings out of apparently nowhere! Physical manifestation of objects is also theoretically possible.

The bizarre behaviour of animals prior to earthquakes,

even before seismological tremors are observable is probably due to unusual scalar wave activity generated by the stressed rock and crystal within the earth's crust, which would naturally build up before its release in an earthquake, animals normally being more sensitive to scalar waves than humans.

As we said, in the context of this theory, earth energies are scalar waves, formed due to both mineral content as well as stress factors in the underlying rocks, many of which are crystalline in nature, and it is a possibility that the highly creative, yet often socially unstable character of Californians is due to the background entrainment through scalar wave resonance in that highly-stressed, earthquake-prone area of the world! It's just an idea!

Interestingly enough, the only scalar wave technology laboratories with which I am familiar are located in California and Japan, another geographical area prone to rock stress and earthquake.

In acupuncture, the use of small magnets, electrical stimulation, hand energies as in acupressure, or the application of mechanical stress with a needle, will all affect the delicate balance of materialization, altering the virtual energy condition at acu-points or wherever applied, since the chakras are seen as major scalar wave resonances within the body, while the nadis and acupuncture meridians represent scalar currents, with particular resonances being located at the acupuncture points.

And so it continues. Many of the phenomena discussed in this book can be described in terms of this new approach. Electromagnetic radiation, being the result of subtle energy substructures, will conversely affect the subtle energy harmony. Chemical pollution in an area will have a tendency to spread by scalar wave transmission, perhaps throughout the whole planet, even though the source of pollution may be isolated, from a chemical point of view.

The substructure of crystals can be mentally programmed to contain information or it may be used simply as a channeling for mental intent. Pulsors are also described as scalar wave resonators through the structuring, sizing, layering and positioning in the thin films of microcrystals of which they consist. Even Keely's failure, mentioned earlier in this chapter, is understandable for his model zeppelin, running of the transformed power of a note from a violin, required the presence not only of Keely's own mental scalar energy, but also the charged-up scalar potential of his laboratory. Without both Keely's presence and the subtle charge of his own place of work, primed by his own thoughts and activity, his experiments would not work.

Radionics is a pure scalar wave science requiring both the intention of the practitioner and the vibration of the witness for its results. And because of the spatio-temporal aspects of scalar wave theory, there is an inherent holographic effect which allow the vibration of a part (the witness) to reflect the nature of the whole.

Morphogenetic fields can be seen as scalar substructures, with the electric gradients of the body as field effects caused by scalar wave activity, while the mind/emotion/body link-up is clearly understandable in energetic terms.

Theoretically, it can be seen that intricate scalar wave substructure engineering can be used to heal or ameliorate illness, within the context of the higher patterning of the individual's karmas. It is often said that energy medicine is the medicine of the future, and the manipulation of the subtle energy fields provides the key to this assertion, while scalar wave technology presents one possible therapeutic methodology.

So the theory is one of tremendous breadth. It also, of course, provides a place for classical mechanics, the known 'laws of nature' and macroscopically observable phenomena. But it is, even so, an outward conceptualization of only the subtle and gross aspects of physical life. It does not, in any way, supplant the spiritual life or provide an understanding of the higher regions of the soul and the inner mystic experience. These are beyond thought, beyond words. If anything, this kind of thinking should provide a spiritual incentive.

Vibrational Science

It can never be repeated often enough that modern technology has, historically, only been prevalent for a fraction of a cosmic second. It has developed and continues to develop at what appears to us to be an amazing pace and yet the basic breakthrough concepts are relatively few in number and well separated in time. The great inventor Nicola Tesla once commented that the difference between himself and Eddison was that he was a true inventor, an originator of new concepts and a builder of altogether new devices, while Eddison was a designer who brilliantly used already existing concepts and applied them in ingenious fashion. It was Tesla, one should add who before the turn of this century conceived, designed, prototyped and tested, *in his own mind*, an entire electrical system, complete with the induction motor, generators, transformers etc, based on alternating current, at a time when Eddison and his direct current generator, motors and light bulbs were considered the only practical approach to the use of electricity. Tesla had the most amazing ability to design his inventions mentally, right down to the last detail and thousandth of an inch. He tested his prototypes mentally, too, which meant that when he finally built his equipment it usually worked first time, with minimal refinements required.

According to Bearden, Tesla also understood intuitively the mechanisms of scalar wave transmission and its relationship to electromagnetism, with Tesla waves being identical to scalar waves. Tesla, in fact, had schemes to put the whole earth into a particular scalar resonance for the "wire-less transmission of energy at a distance", through scalar interferometry effects, but his work was never completed.

Unfortunately, Tesla had no real sense of business and was taken advantage of to such a degree, that although he is regarded by those who know of his work as 'The man who invented the 20th century', even in his own lifetime many did not realize that the fortunes they had made out of practical applications of his alternating current systems were due to his work. Indeed, Tesla, for a time worked for Eddison, improving his direct current systems and designing new equipment, but left in disgust when the promised financial rewards for his work – never committed to paper or made into a legal format – were not forthcoming. Tesla thought electricity. He designed the wireless several years before Marconi introduced it. His ambitious project to build a global wire-less transmitting and receiving station ran out of funds and was dismantled, because Tesla had relinquished the right to a dollar a horsepower royalty for the use of his alternating current patents, in order to help a friend out of financial difficulties. His ideas for the wireless and global transmission of electrical energy, back in the early nineteen hundreds, are concepts which are only now being re-considered by modern scalar electromagnetic and virtual energy theories.

The point is, that although development of numerous devices and sub-theories etc. is rapid once one major new concept is introduced, the frequency with which radically new ways of looking at things are both expounded and accepted is low. I believe that this is because a new concept takes time to mature, to become an integral part of a culture. Moreover, the further we travel down an avenue based on one family of basic concepts, the more difficult it is to step sideways into another way of conceiving or looking at our achievements or areas of mystification.

Thus it is that the ideas expressed in this book may appear to some folk to be new, while others will realize that what is described is, in some respects, no more than a meeting between modern rational science and the ancient wisdom of eastern cultures. It is not so much a challenge, as an adventure; not a confrontation of opposites, but a merging of similarities.

It is necessary to realize that there is indeed no truly objective experience – everything, even our sensory experiences are experienced within ourselves. When we see an object, we think that it is outside. But the light that represents that object is formed by our eye into an inverted image on the retina, becomes an electrical impulse in our optic nerve, is decoded by the brain, the information transformed into more subtle energies where it is appreciated by our physical mind in which our sense of personal ego or identity is lodged, and we feel that we have seen the object. But what makes us so sure that the direction of perception is from the without to the within and not from the within to the without? Do we not feel that we *see* from within? Indeed the great Indian mystic Kabir, back in the fourteenth century, described his own experience thus: 'The inward and the outward have become as one sky.'

This world is the play of karma – cause and effect. What

happens outside *has already happened,* due to our past actions. Our outward life *is already present within us,* awaiting manifestation as our destiny. The seeds have already been sown, the play is already in motion.

Just like the frame-by-frame images in celluloid of a movie picture, the images are transmitted in continuous and exact sequence onto the screen of our outward life. But the audience – ourselves – does not feel that it is a movie. We get involved with the characters and scenes presented to us, identifying with the dream sequences until we feel we are a part of it and that it is real. My own spiritual Master once commented: 'Actually, the problem is that what we see doesn't exist, and what we don't see, really does exist.' The great Hindu goal of detachment from illusion, from Maya, is given a scientific corroboration when physists tell us that what we perceive with our senses, is not what scientific instrumentation perceives. Who has ever seen the dancing, spinning sea of sub-atomic energy that comprises our physical world? None but a few psychics and mystics, considered irrelevant (or worse) by all but a few physicists. If I were a professional physicist and I heard of someone who had actually seen the world of sub-atomic matter and energy, I would want to meet them right away. I'd want to know how they did it, too. But prejudice and ego are a blinding screen even against that which we are seeking to know.

Therefore, we need to be awake to the probability that there will be new scientific concepts put forward that will radically alter our approach to technology as well as our philosophy of life. We must be ready to overcome our mental inertia, our ego, our jealousy and the whole host of unworthy thoughts and emotions that make us so human.

Let us consider, then – and just for fun, if you prefer it – a new approach to all scientific knowledge, an approach I have called: *Vibrational Science.* Vibrational Science I would define as that approach to science which sees the entire cosmos – both 'external' and within living creatures – as a vibrating dance of energy patterns. One's science then consists of an analysis of this dance, lying in the discovery of energy relationships and adequate models, mathematical or otherwise, as appropriate, to enable us to function more effectively – physically, emotionally and mentally within this dance. Our devices or instrumentation (and indeed much of our life) are then seen as nothing more than rearranging the energy patterns, according to our understanding of their interrelationships. This gives us, too, a basis for an ecologically sound approach to science, since no event, device, artifact or human action is seen as separate from the whole cosmos – everything has a relationship to everything else, however tenuous.

However, because it is the easiest way of scientifically analyzing our physical reality, much of present day science has concentrated on observing and identifying discreet objects: things, particles, lumps, molecules, atoms, etc.

Even energy interchanges and forces are reduced to identifiable patterns and wave forms, units of energy – ohms, photons, wavelengths and frequencies, to mention but a few. Once identified and quantified, our neatly pinned (but dead) butterfly can be the subject of mathematics – our language of science – and we are well on the way to a host of inventions and devices. And that's great (partly)!

But look at it for a moment, from a more poetic point of view. Let us add into the melting pot our own subjective experiences of consciousness and being, of beauty and ugliness, with our whole reactive mechanism to the people, living creatures, objects and events that make up our days. We then have our sea of vibrating energy interchange. Human *appreciation* or cognisance of the 'objective' has put us back into the subjective realm of things as we experience them.

All our leading sciences can, I believe, benefit from a re-think along vibrational lines. Modern physics needs to realize even more deeply the fundamental role of motion and polarity as an inherent aspect of energy existence and that energy exists in a vertical, causally creative spectrum, as well as in horizontal, causal relationships. Wave and vibrational patterns and propagation at sub-atomic levels need deeper investigation. Scalar Electromagnetic theory and the whole concept of virtual energy needs considerably more thought, recognition and practical research. Molecular biology needs to consider the existence of its molecules as a vibratory energy complex, including its electronic, magnetic, sub-atomic and subtle states.

In order to build ecologically sound devices, mathematics and engineering need to be able to take into account a vast realm of hitherto unconsidered relationships and subtle oscillatory patterns in order to model more fully the dynamic and interconnected play of energy patterns and pathways. Physiology, anatomy, biology, botany, ecology all need to adopt a more wholistic approach; to understand the vibrational whole in which they are operating, the super-active processes involved in life energies and their reflections at the macroscopic or more easily observable levels where these disciplines operate.

Breadth and vision are required. It is inherently more complex, at the outward level, than present day thinking, but the heart of it is moving towards simplicity and oneness. And one of the results will be a technology and an understanding that leads to a harmony, to a fusion of our personal interests with those of humanity, to a merging of science with a spiritually based philosophy, to a more integrated and wholesome planetary atmosphere.

Epilogue

In the few months, since completing the major part of this book in December 1985 and receiving it back for final adjustments prior to printing, I have received word of many researchers and thinking people around the world who have been working along similar lines with regard especially to the bioelectronic etc., 'information storage' system of our bodies – the non-random meaning in the energy patterns that make up our existence. Some folk might think, 'What a co-incidence!', but this phenomenon of scientific researchers working independently, but coming up with the same results simultaneously is quite widely known. It is reminiscent of the observed phenomenon of similar changes in social, philosophical or moral outlook that seem to arise almost independently in different parts of the world in certain similar sections of the community, but at the same time.

If you observe a wave on the seashore, but give attention only to those parts of the crest which are breaking, then you will see isolated, but similar events happening with apparently inexplicable simultaneity. But if you perceive the wave itself, then you can see that it is an essential part of the energy of the whole event, that it breaks almost simultaneously, separately but not independently, along its length. It is in the nature of things.

This wave – the vibrational and holistic understanding of energy patterns – is just beginning to break. I will be both fascinated and delighted to hear from anyone working or thinking along similar lines. I have other books currently in progress and would like to hear from such pioneers both from personal interest and in case I can help in bringing their work to the attention of a wider public. These are exciting times.

Bibliography and Further Reading

The Aura
The Aura, W.J. Kilner. Originally published as *The Human Atmosphere* (1911); Weiser, 1984.

Aura, How to Read and Understand It, Adelman and Fine; Somaiya, 1981.

The Raiment of Light, David Tansley; Routledge and Kegan Paul, 1984.

Bach Flower Remedies
The Bach Remedies Repertory, F.J.Wheeler; C.W. Daniel, 1985.

Handbook of the Bach Flower Remedies, Philip Chancellor; C.W. Daniel, 1985.

Heal Thyself, Edward Bach; C.W. Daniel; 1985.

Introduction to the Benefits of the Bach Flower Remedies, Jane Evans; C.W. Daniel, 1984.

The Medical Discoveries of Edward Bach,Physician, Nora Weeks; C.W. Daniel, 1973.

The Twelve Healers and Other Remedies, Edward Bach; C.W. Daniel, 1983.

Biomagnetism
Healing by Biomagnetism, Bruce Copen; Academic Publications, 1960.

The Magnetic Blueprint of Life, Davis & Rawls; Exposition Press, 1979.

Magnetism and Its Effects on The Living System, Davis and Rawls; Exposition Press, 1974.

The Magnetic Effect, Davis and Rawls; Exposition Press, 1983.

Magnetic Guidance of Organisms, Richard Frankel. Annual Review of Biophysics and Bioengineering, Vol. 13; Annual Reviews Inc., 1984.

Colour Healing
The Healing Power of Colour, Betty Wood; Thorsons, 1984.

The Seven Keys to Colour Healing, Roland Hunt; C.W. Daniel, 1981.

Dowsing, Radiesthesia and Radionics
Chakras – Rays and Radionics, David Tansley; C.W. Daniel, 1984.

The Chain of Life, Guyon Richards; Speight, 1954.

Divining the Primary Sense, H. Weaver; Routledge & Kegan Paul, 1978.

Dowsing, T. Graves; Thorsons, 1976.

Pendulum Power, Nielsen and Polansky; Thorsons, 1981.

The Power of The Pendulum, T.C. Lethbridge; Routledge and Kegan Paul, 1984.

The Practice of Medical Radiesthesia, Vernon Wethered; C.W. Daniel, 1967.

Radionics & The Subtle Anatomy of Man, David Tansley; C.W. Daniel, 1972.

Earth Energies and Feng Shui
Feng Shui, Sarah Rossbach; Hutchinson, 1983.

Geopathic Stress: The Reason Why Therapies Fail? Anthony Scott-Morley; Journal of Alternative Medicine, May 1985.

Ley Lines, Havelock Fidler; Thorsons, 1983.

New Wave Magnetic Field Therapy, Anthony Scott-Morley; Journal of Alternative Medicine, August 1985.

The Pattern of The Past, Underwood; Pitman, 1969.

Superstrings: A Theory of Everything?, Simon Anthony; New Scientist, August 29, 1985.

Electrical and Electromagnetic Phenomena And Living Creatures

Blueprint for Immortality, Harold S. Burr; Spearman, 1952.

The Cycles of Heaven, Guy Lyon Playfair and Scott Hill; Souvenir, 1978.

Electrographic Imaging in Medicine and Biology, Dumitrescu and Kenyon; Spearman, 1983.

Electromagnetic Fields and Life, A.S. Presman; Plenum, 1970.

Electromagnetism and Life, Robert O. Becker and A. Marino; State University of New York, 1982.

The Menace of Electric Smog, Lowell Ponte; Reader's Digest, U S A., January 1980.

Mind, Body and Electromagnetism, John Evans; Element, 1986.

Mora Therapy: A Revolution in Electro-Magnetic Medicine, Geoffrey Foulkes and Anthony Scott-Morley; Journal of Alternative Medicine, July 1984.

Radiation – What It Is, What It Does To Us & What We Can Do About It, John Davidson M.A. Cantab; C.W. Daniel, 1986.

The Secret of Life, Georges Lakhovsky.

Healing and Subtle Energies

Breakthrough to Certainty, Shafria Karagulla, De Vorss, 1967.

Chakras – Rays and Radionics, David V. Tansley D.C.; C.W. Daniel, 1984.

Esoteric Healing, Alice Bailey; Lucis, 1953.

The Etheric Double, A.E. Powell; Theosophical Publishing House, 1925

Eyewitness to Shamanism, George Sandwith; The Ley Hunter.

Flower Essences and Vibrational Healing, Gurudas and Kevin Ryerson; Brotherhood of Life, 1983.

Healing Energies, Dr Stephen Shepard; Biworld, 1983.

Health Building, The Conscious Art of Living Well, Dr Randolph Stone; CRCS, 1985.

Joy's Way, Brugh Joy; Tarcher, 1979.

Keely and His Discoveries, C.B. Moore; University Books, 1971.

The Odic Force, Karl von Reichenbach; University Books, 1968.

The Orgone Accumulator, Wilhelm Reich; Orgone Institute Press, 1951.

The Pattern of Health, Aubrey Westlake; Shambala, 1973.

Polarity Therapy – Volumes I & II, The Collected Works, Dr Randolph Stone; CRCS, 1986.

The Principles and Art of Cure by Homoeopathy, Herbert A. Roberts M.D.; Health Science Press (now C.W. Daniel), 1979.

The Rainbow in Your Hands, Davis and Rawls; Exposition Press, 1976.

Radionics and The Subtle Anatomy of Man, David V. Tansley D.C., C.W. Daniel, 1972

Miscellaneous

Aboriginal Men of High Degree, A.P. Elkin; University of Queensland, 1977.

The Complete Book of Acupunture, Dr Stephen Chang; Celestial Arts, 1976.

Companion Plants, Dr Helen Philbrick and Gregg; Publisher ??

Green Pharmacy, Barbara Griggs; Norman and Hobhouse, 1982.

A Harmony of Science & Nature – Ways of Staying Healthy in A Modern World, John and Farida Davidson; Wholistic Research Company, 1986.

Introduction to Submolecular Biology, Szent Gyorgi; 1960.

The Life of Nicola Tesla, John J.O'Neil; Spearman, 1968.

The Principles and Art of Cure by Homoeopathy, Herbert A. Roberts M.D., Health Science Press, 1942.

Radiation – What It Is, What It Does To Us & What We Can Do About It, John H. Davidson M.A. Cantab; C.W. Daniel, 1986.

Stalking the Wild Pendulum, Isaac Bentov; Fontana, 1979.

Supernature, Lyall Watson; Coronet, 1983.

The Surgin's Mate, John Woodhall; London, 1617.

The Tao of Physics, Fritjof Capra; Fontana, 1984.

A Treatise of The Scurvy, Jame Lind; Edinburgh, 1953.

Mystic and Yogic Philosophy
Autobiography of a Yogi, Paramhamsa Yogananda; Rider, 1950

The Book Of Mirdad, Anon. Translated by Mikhail Naimy; Clear Press, 1983

The Master Answers, Maharaj Charan Singh Ji; Radha Soami Satsang Beas, 1966.

The Mystic Bible, Dr Randolph Stone; Radha Soami Satsang Beas, 1956.

Mystic Experiences of Medieval Saints, R.P. Aug. Ponlain S.J.; Kegan Paul. Out of Print.

The Path of the Masters, Dr. Julian Johnson; Radha Soami Satsang Beas, 1939.

Spiritual Gems, Maharaj Sawan Singh Ji; Radha Soami Satsang Beas, 1965.

Pulsors and Crystals
Cosmic Crystals, Ra Bonewitz; Thorsons, 1983.

The Crystal Book, Dale Walker; The Crystal Company.

Herbal Crystals as Curative Patterns, George Benner; Private typed manuscript; 1980.

The Magic of Precious Stones, Mellie Uyldert; Thorsons, 1982.

Pulsor, Cosmic Life Force Gyroscope, Dr George Yao; Yao International, 1978.

Pulsor Seminars, Dr George Yao; held in Cambridge 1984 & 1985.

Pulsor, Miracle of Micro-Crystals, Dr George Yao & Thomas Bearden; Gyro Industries, 1986.

Pyramids
The Guide to Pyramid Energy, Kerrell and Goggin; Force, 1975.

Pyramid Power, Dr Pat Flanagan; De Vorss, 1973.

Pyramid Power, Toth & Nielsen; Destiny Books, 1985.

Pyramid Power and Psychic Healing, Graydon Dixon; Pythagorean Press, 1978.

Index

Further Information

Many of the books and products mentioned herein, including Pulsors®, are available from the:

WHOLISTIC RESEARCH COMPANY
Bright Haven,
Robin's Lane,
Lolworth,
Cambridge CB3 8HH,
England.

Telephone: Craft's Hill (0954) 81074

Please send £1.95 (£4.00 overseas), for their large and full information pack, including their 72pp book/catalogue: *A Harmony Of Science & Nature – Ways Of Staying Healthy In A Modern World,* by John & Farida Davidson.

Training in the use of Pulsors® and in understanding subtle energy is given by the author, contactable through the above address. Visits, by appointment only, please.